Brain Fluids and Metabolism

BRAIN FLUIDS
AND METABOLISM

Gary A. Rosenberg, M.D.

University of New Mexico School of Medicine
and the Neurology Service,
Veterans Medical Center
Albuquerque, New Mexico

New York   Oxford
OXFORD UNIVERSITY PRESS
1990

Oxford University Press

Oxford   New York   Toronto
Delhi   Bombay   Calcutta   Madras   Karachi
Petaling Jaya   Singapore   Hong Kong   Tokyo
Nairobi   Dar es Salaam   Cape Town
Melbourne   Auckland
and associated companies in
Berlin   Ibadan

Library of Congress Cataloging-in-Publication Data
Rosenberg, Gary A.
Brain fluids and metabolism/Gary A. Rosenberg.
p.   cm. Includes index. ISBN 0-19-505324-9
1. Cerebrospinal fluid.   2. Brain—Metabolism.
3. Cerebral edema.   4. Cerebral ischemia.
I. Title. [DNLM:
1. Brain—Metabolism.   2. Cerebrospinal Fluid—metabolism.
WL 203 R813b] QP375.R67   1990 612.8'2—dc20
DNLM/DLC   for Library of Congress   89-16140   CIP

9 8 7 6 5 4 3 2 1
Printed in the United States of America
on acid-free paper

To
Evelyn
Oren
And
Mica

Preface

The practice of neurology is undergoing dramatic upheavals. Technological breakthroughs in electronic sensors, computer technology, and isotope detection have produced a series of new instruments that have made it possible to visualize brain structures to millimeter resolution and to analyze brain metabolism noninvasively. Once relegated entirely to the world of pure research, these technological advances are encroaching more and more into the decisions we make daily in the care of patients. Parallel with the advances in clinical neurosciences there has been an explosion of information in the basic neurosciences. The number of neurotransmitters and neuromodulators continues to grow, electrical signals from ion channels can be recorded, and genetic loci for inherited illnesses have been found—to name but a few of the areas in which our understanding has been increased. For the neurologist and neuroscientist, it is important to understand the place of this information in relation to problems that arise in the care of patients, but access to this information is complicated by its technical nature and the scattered places in which it is published.

For the past several years, I have given the medical students and the housestaff of the University of New Mexico School of Medicine lectures on brain fluids and metabolism. Initially, the emphasis was on cerebrospinal fluid and brain edema because that had the most clinical relevance. More recently, however, the lectures have included information on PET scanning, MRI, and other new methods to study brain function. These topics fell together under brain metabolism and offered insights into the physiological changes on a molecular level. This material is unavailable in a form accessible to clinicians, and for that reason I have organized these lectures into a short textbook.

This will of necessity be a personal view, looking more closely at things that I have done and giving less emphasis to other areas in which I am less familiar. The broad range of topics covered will lead to errors in some areas, particularly those in which information is still being gathered. Every effort has been made to find and remove such errors.

The book is loosely organized into three parts. The first part gives an overview of the book in Chapter 1 and describes the anatomy in Chapter 2 and the physiology in Chapter 3 of the brain fluids or so-called third circulation, which will be important for understanding Chapter 9 on brain edema. The second part has more technical material. It covers the areas of molecular transport in Chapter 4, autoradiograms and PET scans in Chapter 5, and the fundamentals of biological nuclear magnetic resonance in Chapter 6. The second part forms the basis for understanding Chapter 7 on normal transport and metabolism and Chapter 8 on energy failure.

The book was begun during a sabbatical stay with Professor Michael Bradbury at King's College, London. The work from our laboratory has been supported by grants from the March of Dimes, the American Heart Association, the Veterans Administration, and the National Institutes of Health.

I have been fortunate to have worked in the past and at present with individuals with insights into the neurological sciences. Dr. Robert Katzman stimulated my interest in brain edema and hydrocephalus. Others who have shaped my thinking include Drs. Leslie Wolfson, Clifford Patlak, Joseph Fenstermacher, Ronald Blasberg, and Helen Cserr. My close association with Edward Estrada and Dr. Walter Kyner over many years has been invaluable. Dr. Jim Brainard helped me to appreciate NMR. My colleagues in New Mexico Drs. Jim Brainard, Mario Kornfeld, Fred Mettler, Jr., Linda Saland, and Gaynor Wild provided illustrations and suggestions. The permission from various publishers to use illustrations from their journals and textbooks is greatly appreciated. Alisa Sherwood prepared the manuscript, and the Oxford editor, Dr. Alasdair Ritchie, worked closely with me on the final text.

G.A.R.

Albuquerque
January 1990

Contents

Brain Fluids and Metabolism

1

Fluids, Circulation, and Metabolism:
An Overview

1.1 INTRODUCTION

In the past 10 years, the practice of neurology has undergone dramatic changes in large part because of the development of new tools. Structural details of brain pathology have become available with computed tomography (CT) and magnetic resonance imaging (MRI). The pathophysiology of stroke, epilepsy, dementia, and Parkinson's disease has been investigated using position emission tomography (PET). Nuclear magnetic resonance spectroscopy (NMR) has been used to study brain metabolism. Electromagnetic changes have been studied with evoked responses and more recently with magnetoencephalography. CT and MRI have aided greatly our ability to diagnose diseases and to localize pathological changes. PET and NMR have helped us understand the underlying pathophysiology of several diseases and may affect treatment in the future. Interpretation of the results of these tests requires an understanding of the physiology and chemistry of the nervous system.

The clinical neurological examination demonstrates dysfunction of specific parts of the nervous system. By observing the results of different tests, the site of abnormal function generally can be determined, a diagnosis of the underlying pathophysiology made, and a plan of treatment devised. Neurologists of the late nineteenth and early twentieth centuries by bedside examination and subsequent pathological correlation described a large number of neurological syndromes. Their understanding of the underlying pathophysiology of the disease states was very limited, however, and treatments for most illnesses were either empirical or, in many cases, nonexistent.

In the past 50 years, the complex nature of nervous tissue has been un-

3

raveled with electron microscopy, biochemical analysis, and neurophysiological studies. This has resulted in a more complete understanding of fluid dynamics, cerebral circulation, and neurotransmission. By analysis of the parts of the nervous system separately, the function of individual components has been determined. This has been done by cell culture methods to study homogeneous cell types, single cell recording of electrical events, isolation of cerebral vessels for permeability studies, and so on. Integration of this information has provided a picture of nervous tissue function.

The whole is greater than the sum of its parts, and although much is known about each individual component, the function of the whole brain cannot be explained. Therefore, the ability to analyze brain function in living organisms by electroencephalography (EEG), PET, NMR, and other methods is of great importance.

Nervous tissue is composed of neurons, astrocytes, glial, ependymal, pial, and endothelial cells, and connecting tissues. Blood passing through brain tissue is separated from these cells by a series of interfaces, with tight junctions between cells. The fluid environment of the nervous system is very closely regulated by the secretion of cerebrospinal and interstitial fluids, which perform a lymph-like function for the brain. Passage of substances from the blood to the brain across the capillary is the major route of delivery of glucose and oxygen to the cells. Analysis of the blood–brain barrier, which had been limited to the laboratory, can now be performed in patients with CT and MRI, using contrast agents. In addition, measurements of cerebral blood flow and metabolism, which formerly were extremely difficult to perform and required both intracarotid injections and sampling of venous blood at the jugular bulb, are carried out using PET and NMR, making these measurements less traumatic.

With the recent introduction into clinical practice of procedures previously used only in a few laboratories, it is necessary for the clinician to understand the underlying physiology. Interpretation of the results of these tests involves understanding the circulation of cerebrospinal and interstitial fluid, the transport of nutrients into the central nervous system (CNS), and the metabolism of these nutrients by brain cells, with the production of metabolic products. Complex changes are associated with breakdown of brain cells. The new diagnostic methods show the dynamic changes occurring as the tissue is damaged. This new information should provide the basis for more specific treatments.

1.2. HISTORICAL SURVEY

Our knowledge of the brain dates back to ancient times. Many early concepts have been replaced as new information has become available. However, some of the early concepts have persisted, and the original insights are still accepted.

The ancient Greeks knew of the ventricles in the brain but did not realize they contained fluid. Galen (130–200 AD), who described the cavities in the brain, thought they were filled with a vapor. He also thought that nasal catarrh arose from the brain. Andreas Vesalius (1514–1564), the great Italian anatomist, accurately drew the cerebral ventricles. The first physiologic studies were carried out by Richard Lower (1631–1691) at Oxford; he showed that nasal catarrh was nothing more than nasal secretion. Lower wrote that the brain fluids arose from the arterial supply and drained into the venous system. He was the first to divorce the intraventricular fluid from ancient vitalism and to recognize it as a watery fluid "similar to lymph" (Brisman, 1970).

Domenico Cotugno (1736–1822), professor of surgery and anatomy at the University of Naples, discovered that the ventricles were filled with the cerebrospinal fluid (CSF) in life. He discovered this by performing autopsies on cadavers before severing the head from the body, the normal custom that allowed the fluid to drain away before the skull was opened (Levinson, 1936). Another major advance was made by Gustaf Retzius (1842–1919), who showed that the pacchionian bodies of the cerebral venous sinuses were the site of drainage of CSF into blood. Heinrich Quincke (1842–1922) introduced the lumbar puncture into clinical practice in 1891 and was the first to use it as a method to remove fluid in children with hydrocephalus. He also described the effect of diseases on the CSF. Hans Queckenstedt (1876–1918) developed a test for spinal fluid obstruction in 1916. It is based on the fact that during a lumbar puncture, compression of the jugular veins results in a rapid rise in the CSF pressure to over twice the normal value, which returns rapidly to normal after release of the jugular compression. If a spinal block is present, the pressure fall occurs much more slowly. This test is rarely used clinically at this time.

The modern era of spinal fluid studies was begun in the late nineteenth century by Mott, Weed, and Cushing. Lewis Weed, working in the laboratory of Harvey Cushing, formulated the concept that interstitial fluid originated from cerebral capillaries, forming a lymphatic system for brain (Weed, 1914). Harvey Cushing used the term "the Third Circulation" to emphasize the importance of both the cerebrospinal and interstitial fluids in normal brain function. Blood was the first circulation, lymph the second, and brain fluids the third. This was a true circulation, with formation of CSF in the choroid plexus and drainage back into the blood (Figure 1–1). Cushing summarized the work of Weed and his colleagues from the Hunterian Laboratory at Johns Hopkins (Cushing, 1925). He clearly understood the need for a fluid system in nervous tissue when he wrote: "Are there lymph channels in the brain, and if not, how does the central nervous system dispose of its products of tissue waste?" Weed referred to the perivascular space of Virchow and Robin as a series of channels carrying fluid from the brain to the subarachnoid space (Weed, 1914).

The concept of the blood–brain barrier came from studies by Ehrlich and Goldmann (Bradbury, 1979). Ehrlich, in 1885, showed that a dye injected into the blood stained all organs except the brain. Goldmann, in 1913, found

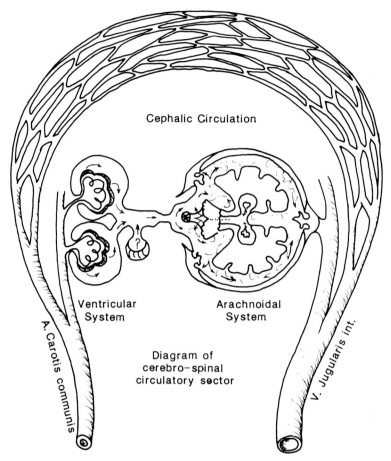

Cephalic Circulation

Ventricular   Arachnoidal
System   System

A. Carotis communis

V. Jugularis int.

Diagram of
cerebro-spinal
circulatory sector

Figure 1–1. Diagram of the CSF circulation from choroid plexus to the arachnoid villi. (From Cushing, 1925)

that trypan blue dye injected into the CSF did stain brain tissue. These two simple experiments were sufficient to show that a barrier existed between blood and brain and that a substance in the CSF had access to brain tissue.

In spite of physiological evidence for the presence of an extracellular space for the interstitial fluid to flow through the brain, ultrastructural studies in the 1950s using the electron microscope failed to show a space. Since the extracellular space could not be found, anatomists and physiologists postulated that the glial cells regulated fluid and electrolytes. The glial transport theory persisted until 1962, when Rall et al. (1962) analyzed the diffusion patterns of extracellular molecules during ventriculocisternal perfusion. They found that extracellular space comprises about 15–20 percent of the brain. Anatomical confirmation followed when improved methods of tissue fixation showed an extracellular space at the ultrastructural level (Van Harreveld and Khattub, 1969).

Advances in our understanding of brain metabolism also have been recent. Kety and Schmidt (1945) were the first to measure cerebral blood flow in humans by arteriovenous differences for inhaled nitrous oxide. Kety (1950) based his measurements on the Fick principle, which measures flow to an organ by the amount of dilution of an inert tracer. By this method, oxygen consumption and glucose utilization rates in whole brain have been measured in a variety of disease states, including stroke, dementia, and schizophrenia. Lowry and Passonneau (1964) were the first to completely characterize the substrates and enzymes involved in carbohydrate metabolism in animals, whereas the neurochemistry of lipids was explored by Folch-Pi et al. (1957). In the years since these pioneering studies in blood flow, metabolism, and chemical composition, enormous amounts of information have been gathered, extending our understanding of brain function.

1.3. BRAIN-FLUID INTERFACES

Extensive studies of the anatomy of the brain, particularly at the interfaces between brain tissue and the systemic circulation, have resulted in a view of brain tissue as an organ isolated in many ways from the circulation. This separation is necessary to ensure that the fluids bathing the brain cells have a well-regulated chemical composition.

The brain microenvironment is controlled by a series of interfaces between the brain tissue and the systemic fluids (Figure 1–2). Neurons require a

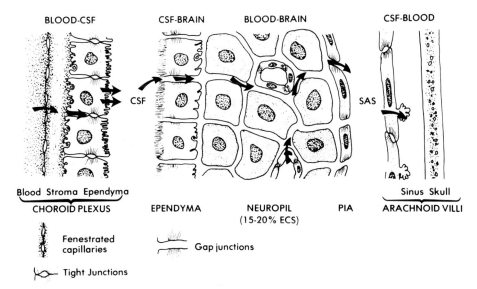

Figure 1–2. Schematic diagram of interfaces between blood, brain, and CSF. Arrows indicate formation of CSF at the choroid plexus and interstitial fluid (ISF) at the brain capillary. The CSF-ISF is absorbed into blood at the arachnoid villi. ECS, extracellular space; SAS, subarachnoid space. (From Rosenberg et al., 1983)

consistent ionic composition in the extracellular space and are much less tolerant of changes than are other cells (Davson, 1967; Katzman and Pappius, 1973). Therefore, substances that circulate in the blood in fluctuating concentrations are excluded from the brain. This helps to prevent wide fluctuations in electrolytes in brain fluids. As a result, the CSF has a well-regulated ionic composition in contact with the interstitial fluid.

Three interfaces in the CNS separate the brain from the systemic circulation; they are the capillary endothelial cells, the epithelial cells of the choroid plexus, and the arachnoid (Table 1–1). Within the brain, the ependyma and pia form a fourth interface between the CSF and the brain. The most extensive interface occurs at the blood–brain barrier because of the large surface area of the cerebral capillaries. At each interface where brain cells come into contact with blood there are tight junctions, which are formed when cell surfaces are continuously apposed to one another, preventing movement of nonlipid soluble substances. Epithelial cells vary in their tightness. At one extreme, very tightly joined cells act like membrane sheets (Rapoport, 1976). Gap junctions, on the other hand, are less restrictive because of openings (gaps) in the matrix joining the surfaces. These are found at the internal interfaces between brain and CSF, formed by the ependyma and pia.

The choroid plexuses form the majority of the CSF and are outpocketings of the epithelial cells that line the ventricles. The overlying ependymal cells of the choroid plexus function as a barrier to the free entry of electrolytes and proteins from the blood. However, the ependyma overlying the gray and white matter does not function as a barrier. Hence, once electrolytes and protein are in the CSF, there is little resistance to movement into the brain. Therefore, intrathecal or direct injection into the spinal CSF space provides access to brain tissue for substances normally excluded by the blood–brain barrier. Finally, the arachnoid has tight junctions that prevent exchange of substances in the CSF with the blood. Arachnoid villi are valve-like outpocketings that penetrate the dura at the venous sinuses to drain CSF into blood.

The interfaces are important in normal brain function. The blood–brain interfaces, as a group, serve the basic function of maintaining an ionic composition in the brain fluids for normal neuronal action. Neuronal membranes are particularly sensitive to changes in potassium, calcium, and magnesium. Sodium is important in osmotic balance. Small amounts of protein are allowed to enter brain, but most proteins are prevented from entering brain

Table 1–1. Interfaces Separating Blood from Brain Tissue

Interface	Cell Type	Junction Type
Blood–brain	Endothelial	Tight Junction
Blood–CSF	Epithelium of choroid plexus	Apical tight junction
CSF–blood	Arachnoid cells and villi	Valves in villi; tight junctions in arachnoid
CSF–brain	Ependyma and pia	Gap junctions

cells, and potentially toxic substances are prevented from entering the brain. A series of selective carriers and ion pumps is situated on the interface cells to transport electrolytes and essential nutrients. Blood products toxic to brain tissue, such as bilirubin and lactate, are excluded. The composite of these permissive and exclusive functions has been termed loosely the blood–brain barrier.

1.4. CEREBRAL METABOLISM AND BLOOD FLOW

The brain requires a continuous supply of glucose and oxygen to meet its energy requirements (Sokoloff, 1981). Cerebral oxygen consumption is about 3.5 ml/100 g brain/minute, or, for an average brain of 1,400 g, about 49 ml oxygen per minute. Although the brain represents 2 percent of total body weight, it accounts for 20 percent of the resting total body oxygen consumption.

Glucose and oxygen must be supplied continuously to the brain (Siesjo, 1976). When blood flow to the brain stops, the absence of oxygen and blood results in the loss of consciousness in 5–10 seconds, and if the blood flow is not resumed within several minutes, there is permanent brain damage. The absence of glucose is equally destructive, but the time course to irreversible damage from hypoglycemia is longer because other substrates can be used.

Glucose enters the glycolytic pathways, where it is converted to pyruvate and then metabolized through the Krebs cycle. In anoxic conditions, it is converted into lactate (Figure 1–3). The amounts of glucose (and its storage form glycogen) stored in the brain are small and can be depleted rapidly. In the absence of glucose, the brain uses amino acids and fatty acids, ultimately metabolizing nutrients and membranes causing permanent cell damage. During starvation, ketone bodies are metabolized in place of glucose. Glucose and amino acids are transported across the blood–brain barrier by carrier-mediated systems. These transport systems ensure that the brain has adequate amounts of glucose and amino acids to maintain normal function.

An analog of glucose, 2-deoxyglucose (2-DG), has been used to measure glucose metabolism in experimental animals with autoradiography. 2-Deoxyglucose is transported across the blood–brain barrier by the glucose carrier system and is metabolized in glycolysis through phosphorylation by hexokinase (Sokoloff, 1981). Phosphatase activity has been detected in brain. Because phosphatase can metabolize deoxyglucose, correction for 2-DG metabolism is necessary for quantitation of glucose metabolism by this method. The 2-DG method has been modified for human use with PET, with short-lived positron-emitting isotopes labeled to the 2-DG. Glucose also has been labeled with positron emitters and followed by PET scanning.

The supply of oxygen and glucose to brain tissue depends on the cerebral blood flow. Normally, cerebral blood flow is maintained at a constant level over a wide range of blood pressures by an autoregulatory mechanism, al-

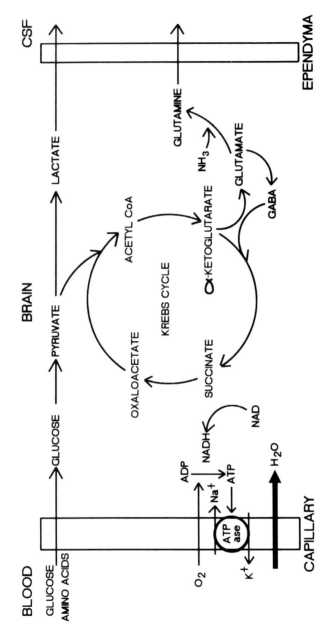

Figure 1–3. Coupling of glucose and oxygen transport to chemiosmotic work and metabolism. Glycolysis in brain cells converts glucose into pyruvate. Under aerobic conditions, the Krebs cycle forms NADH for conversion of ADP to ATP in the respiratory chain. Glutamate can be stored or converted into GABA or glutamine. The action of the Na^+,K^+-ATPase pump is maintained by ATP. Water enters cells down osmotic and hydrostatic gradients.

though at the extremes of blood pressure, the mechanism fails. Hypotension then leads to a fall in cerebral blood flow, and hypertension causes an increase in blood flow, with a breakdown of the blood–brain barrier (Lassen, 1974).

Blood flow was initially measured by the Fick principle using nitrous oxide arteriovenous differences in whole brain (Kety and Schmidt, 1945). Regional measurements of blood flow have been made in humans with a gamma-emitting form of an inert gas, whose clearance from brain can be followed with multiple arrays of radioactivity detectors (Lassen et al., 1963). Blood flow and glucose consumption can be measured with PET scanners. Other information available from PET includes oxygen consumption and receptor binding. PET scanning has been used to study patients with seizures, stroke, dementia, and Parkinson's disease.

Oxygen and other lipid-soluble gases diffuse across the cerebral capillary. When there is no oxygen (anoxia) or blood flow stops (ischemia), the brain switches over to anaerobic metabolism. Lactate is formed, and the brain pH becomes dangerously low. Anaerobic metabolism depletes the brain of essential amino acids and forms excessive amounts of GABA, an inhibitory amino acid. Furthermore, the production of NADH and ATP ceases, which, in turn, means that energy-dependent membrane pumps cannot maintain the chemical and osmotic balance of the brain. Other vital biosynthetic activities also are inhibited.

As the brain's energy substrates are depleted, degradative enzymes are activated, and phospholipases release free fatty acids from the membrane. Arachidonic acid, a free fatty acid, is converted to toxic free radicals in the presence of residual oxygen and irreversibly disrupts the membrane (Raichle, 1983; Siesjo, 1984).

Phosphorus-containing compounds provide energy for the brain. The energy state of the brain is dependent on the levels of phosphocreatine and ATP. As brain failure occurs, there is a loss of phosphocreatine initially, followed by ATP depletion, which generally signals severe damage to the cell. The concentration of ATP can be estimated using NMR spectroscopy. The energy state of large regions of tissue has been monitored by NMR in animals and in humans.

Advances in technology have been faster in the past decade then in the previous 70 years and have made possible analysis during life of brain structure and function (Figure 1–4). CT is an x-ray method of visualizing brain structures with millimeter resolution. Bone is seen clearly because of the calcium it contains, but it produces artifacts in tissues of nearby brain regions. Imaging with MRI is possible because protons in water molecules have magnetic moments. The anatomical detail of MRI is greater than that of CT, particularly next to bone, as in the posterior fossa. However, MRI lacks the ability to show blood and calcium in brain as well as CT.

In addition to new structural information, these technological advances have improved our understanding of the pathophysiology underlying many diseases of the nervous system. These advances have been made because of

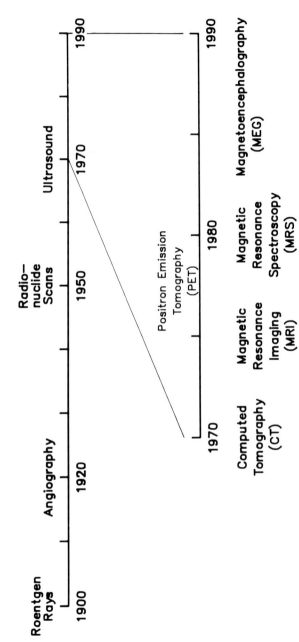

Figure 1–4. The major technological advances in neurodiagnostic procedures in this century.

the application of electron microscopy in anatomy, transport analysis in physiology, and, more recently, NMR in the physical chemistry of cerebral metabolism.

The role of the new diagnostic modalities in clinical practice remains to be determined. Careful evaluation of possible applications by unbiased observers is needed. Often the initial enthusiasm for a new method causes an overzealous evaluation of its usefulness. Therefore, it is important to understand the theoretical basis for the techniques that have potential clinical applications. However, even if their clinical application is limited, the information gained already from PET and NMR has added to our understanding of brain function. Dramatic recent progress has occurred in the long history of neuroscience research, and the rapid increase in knowledge about the brain will most likely continue.

REFERENCES

Bradbury, M. W. B.: *The Concept of a Blood–Brain Barrier.* Chichester; England: John Wiley and Sons, 1979.

Brisman, R.: Pioneer studies on the circulation of the cerebrospinal fluid with particular reference to studies by Richard Lower in 1669. J. Neurosurg. 32:1–4, 1970.

Cushing, H.: *The Third Circulation.* London: Oxford University Press, 1925.

Davson, H.: *Physiology of the Cerebrospinal Fluid.* London: J & A Churchill, 1967.

Folch-Pi, J., Lees M., Sloane-Stanley, G. H.: A simple method for the isolation and purification of total lipids from animal tissues. J. Biol. Chem. 226:497–509, 1957.

Katzman, R., Pappius, H. M.: *Brain Electrolytes and Fluid Metabolism.* Baltimore: Williams & Wilkins Co., 1973.

Kety, S. S.: Circulation and metabolism of the human brain in health and disease. Am. J. Med. 8:205–217, 1950.

Kety, S. S., Schmidt, C. F.: The determination of cerebral blood flow in man by the use of nitrous oxide in low concentrations. Am. J. Physiol. 143:52–66, 1945.

Lassen, N. A.: Control of cerebral circulation in health and disease. Circ. Res. 34:749–760, 1974.

Lassen, N. A., Hoedt-Rasmussen K., Sorensen, S. C., et al.: Regional cerebral blood flow in man determined by krypton. Neurology 13:719–727, 1963.

Levinson A.: Domenico Contugno. Ann. Med. His. 8:1–9, 1936.

Lowry, O. H., Passonneau J. V.: The relationship between substrates and enzymes of glycolysis in brain. J. Biol. Chem. 239:31–32, 1964.

Raichle, M. E.: The pathophysiology of brain ischemia. Ann. Neurol. 13:2–10, 1983.

Rall, D. P., Oppelt, W. W., Patlak, C. S.: Extracellular space of brain as determined by diffusion of inulin from the ventricular system. Life Sci. 1:43–48, 1962.

Rapoport, S. I.: *Blood–Brain Barrier in Physiology and Medicine.* New York: Raven Press, 1976.

Rosenberg, G. A., Wolfson, L. I., Katzman, R.: Disorders of cerebrospinal fluid circulation. In *The Clinical Neurosciences* (Rosenberg, R. N., ed.) Churchill Livingstone, New York: 1983, pp. I:285–300.

Siesjo, B. K.: *Brain Energy Metabolism*. Chichester, England: John Wiley and Sons, 1976.

Siesjo, B. K.: Cerebral circulation and metabolism. J. Neurosurg 60:883–908, 1984.

Sokoloff, L.: Circulation and energy metabolism of the brain. In *Basic Neurochemistry*. Siegel, G. T., Albers, R. W., Agranoff, B. W., Katzman, R., eds. Boston: Little, Brown and Company, 1981:471–495.

Van Harreveld, A., Khattub, F. I.: Changes in extracellular space of the mouse cerebral cortex during hydroxyadipaldehyde fixation and osmium tetroxide post-fixation. J. Cell. Sci. 4:437–453, 1969.

Weed, L. H.: Studies on cerebrospinal fluid. IV. The dual source of cerebrospinal fluid. J Med Res 31:93–117, 1914.

2

Anatomy of Brain Interfaces

2.1 INTRODUCTION

Brain cell survival depends on a carefully regulated fluid environment. Just as the skull provides the barrier to the outside world, the interfaces between blood and brain buffer the inner world. When the barriers separating the blood from the brain are injured, toxic substances from the blood invade the brain. Brain tissue responds poorly to injury. It has delicate membranes, high energy needs for transport and metabolism, and little regenerative potential. Eighty percent of the gray matter is water, and 15 percent of brain tissue is extracellular space. When injury occurs, the water shifts from one compartment to another along osmotic and hydrostatic gradients, which disrupts cellular function and damages vital structures.

The movement of molecules from blood to brain is regulated at a series of interfaces formed by epithelial and arachnoid cells that are tightly joined together to form a series of epithelial sheets. The epithelial cells lining the ventricles and covering the brain are joined by junctions that allow exchange to occur. However, the epithelium of the choroid plexuses and the capillaries restrict exchange (except for lipid-soluble substances that can cross the membrane directly).

Immediately beneath the skull is the dura, a tough membrane that is an important structure that prevents spread of infection from the skull into the brain and contains the CSF. Tears in the dura can occur when the skull is fractured or during neurosurgery. Once the dura is damaged, the CSF can leak out. This leads to symptoms from low CSF pressure or from the introduction of infection into the CNS. Beneath the dura is the arachnoid, whose cells are joined together by tight junctions. The CSF is in the subarachnoid space and is contiguous with the pial cells covering the brain surface. In brain injury, the potential space between the dura and arachnoid can become the site of a subdural hematoma from a ruptured venous blood vessel. Occasionally, an artery between the skull and dura is injured, and an epidural hematoma is formed.

Drainage of CSF occurs across the specialized epithelium of the arachnoid villi and into the lymphatic system. The arachnoid membrane beneath the dura has tight junctions and is an important interface between blood and brain. At specialized regions in the arachnoid membrane where the arachnoid cells overlay the sagittal sinus, the arachnoid cells protrude into the sagittal sinuses to form the arachnoid granulations. These are the sites where CSF drains by a one-way valve mechanism into the blood. In addition, in certain species it appears that a significant proportion of CSF drains along extracellular channels into the lymphatics. However, the importance of the anatomical connections between the brain's extracellular fluids and the extracerebral lymphatics is still unresolved for higher mammals.

2.2 DEVELOPMENT OF BRAIN–FLUID INTERFACES

The nervous system develops from a region in the middorsal line of the embryo. A thickened plate of ectoderm folds in to form the neural groove, which, once closed, becomes the neural tube (Figure 2–1). The cephalic part begins to dilate to form the brain and ventricular system, while the caudal segment that will be the spinal cord maintains a uniform diameter. An internal limiting membrane on the inner surface forms next to the cells that will become the ependyma. At the outer surface is mesenchyma that is separated from the ectoderm by an external limiting membrane. Germinal cells are found between the inner and outer membranes. The mantle layer becomes the gray matter, composed of glia and neurons, and the marginal layer becomes white matter. Ciliated epithelial cells line the neural tube, and cilia persist in some regions of the adult human ependyma.

The neural tube is formed from neuroepithelial cells that extend from the internal to the external limiting membranes (Langman et al., 1966). Nuclei synthesizing DNA are found near the external limiting membrane and migrate toward the inner limiting membrane (Figure 2–2). Once DNA synthesis is over, these cells become the neuroblasts that form the mantle layer. When neuroblasts mature into the neuronal cells of the adult, they lose their ability to divide. Neurons establish synapses with specific nuclear groups probably on the basis of chemical affinities (Figure 2–3). After neuroblast differentiation has ceased, future glial cells are formed from neuroepithelial cells that have differentiated with glioblasts. Ependymal cells are formed along with glioblasts. Ependymal cells and subependymal cells form a separate unit loosely attached to the outer limiting membrane (Carpenter and Sutin, 1983).

The choroid plexuses are formed in specialized regions where underlying blood vessels grow and push out the ependyma. Mesenchyme outside the

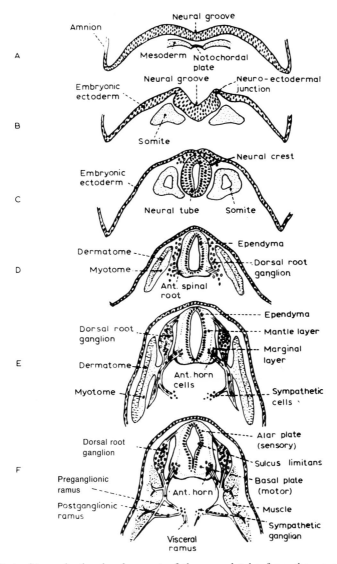

Figure 2–1. Stages in the development of the neural tube from the neural plate, with subsequent formation of spinal cord. (From Schade and Ford, 1965)

outer limiting membrane condenses to become the periosteum, dura, and arachnoid. Fine trabeculi join the arachnoid to the pia, and CSF fills the space between the two membranes. The dura thickens into a tough connective tissue, and the space between the dura and arachnoid is absent except in pathological situations.

Development of the cerebral capillaries depends on trophic factors secreted by brain tissue. Proof that the brain has trophic factors that determine

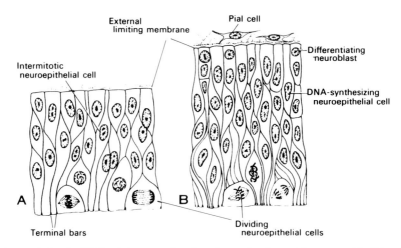

Figure 2–2. A. Wall of the recently closed neural tube, with neuroepithelial cells that form a pseudostratified epithelium extending from the lower to the external limiting membrane. B. Cross-section of the wall of the neural tube at a more advanced stage than in A. Neuroepithelial cells are in phases of DNA synthesis or mitosis, except near the external limiting membrane, where differentiating neuroblasts are found. (From Carpenter and Sutin, 1983)

the type of vessel formed comes from elegant transplant experiments between quail and chick embryos. Transplantation of quail brain into embryonic chick cultures resulted in the formation of systemic vessels, whereas nonbrain tissue transplanted into embryonic brain produced capillaries with tight junctions (Stewart and Wiley, 1981).

Failure of neural tube closure in the first trimester of embryonic life results in congenital anomalies. Dysraphism refers to a group of congenital malformations in which there is failure of the posterior part of the neural tube to close (Gabriel, 1974). Failure of posterior closure produces developmental disorders that range from spina bifida occulta, an incidental finding discovered on routine spinal x-ray, to myelodysplasia, a severe deformation that involves failure of closure of both the midline structures in the posterior fossa of the brain and central canal of the spinal cord and can lead to death. Commonly encountered dysraphic syndromes include absence of cerebral hemisphere development (anencephaly), failure of vertebra and skull to close (spina bifida and cranium bifidum), and the combined spinal and nervous tissue abnormalities of the Chiari malformations. In Chiari type I malformation, there is a protrusion of an elongated cerebellar tonsil into the foramen magnum. When these patients begin to have symptoms, which is usually in adult life, they have signs of lower brainstem dysfunction. Type II Chiari patients have meningomyelocele, and hydrocephalus often is present at birth or becomes manifest when the spinal defect is repaired. Chiari type III and type IV malformations are more extensive malformations of the cerebellum and brainstem and are generally incompatible with life.

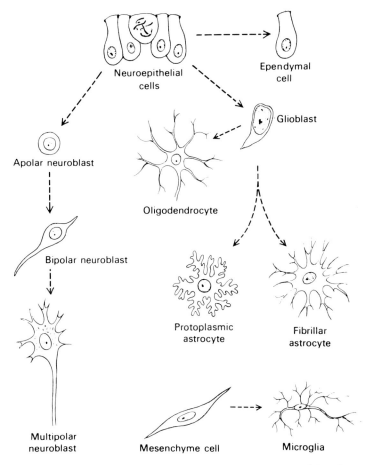

Figure 2–3. Diagram of the histogenesis of neurons and neuroglial cells. Neuro-blasts, glioblasts, and ependymal cells originate from neuroepithelial cells. The or-igin of the oligodendrocyte is obscure, but both protoplasmic and fibrillary astrocytes are derived from glioblasts. The microglia are considered to arise from mesenchyme. (From Carpenter and Sutin, 1983)

2.3 BRAIN–CSF INTERFACE

Cerebrospinal fluid comes into contact with brain cells at the cerebral ven-tricles and over the brain's surface. The exchange of substances between the CSF and the interstitial fluid (ISF) is relatively unrestricted across both the ependymal cells of the ventricle and the pial cells of the surface. Both of these interfaces are formed by epithelial cells with leaky or gap junctions. Brightman and Reese (1969) showed by electron microscopy that the large protein molecule, horseradish peroxidase (HRP), crosses from the CSF into brain extracellular fluid.

The cerebral ventricles enlarge as the brain elongates and enfolds to as-sume its adult shape. In the fully developed brain, the cerebral ventricles are divided anatomically into two lateral ventricles with frontal and occipital poles and the temporal extension. The third ventricle is in the midline between the thalamic nuclei and the hypothalamus, and it is connected to the fourth ventricle by the aqueduct of Sylvius. The ventricles connect with the subarachnoid space in the fourth ventricle through the foramina of Magendie and Luschka (Figure 2–4).

The ventricular surface and choroid plexuses are lined by a heterogeneous

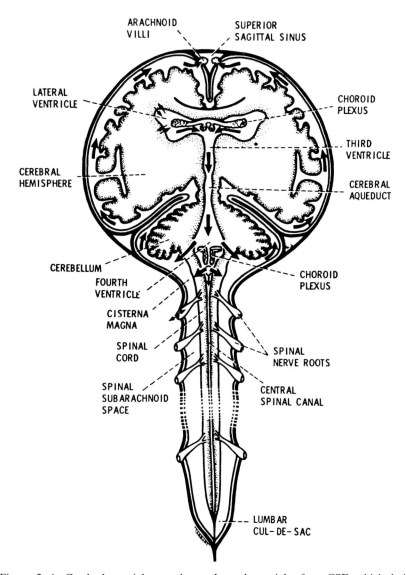

Figure 2–4. Cerebral ventricles are shown. Lateral ventricles form CSF, which drains into the third ventricle through the aqueduct into the fourth. CSF leaves the ventricles at the foramina of Luschka and Magendie. (From Millen and Woollam, 1962)

layer of epithelial cells. Over the choroid plexuses, the epithelial cells are cuboidal in shape and have microvilli on the apical surface next to the CSF. Microvilli are short protrusions from the surface of the cells that increase the surface area. Choroid plexus epithelial cells have nuclei in the basal region, a large number of mitochondria in the cytoplasm, and a high energy requirement. Their apical surfaces are joined by tight junctions. These cells have features in common with those in the kidney that are also involved in active transport (Tennyson and Pappas, 1968).

The ventricular surface overlying brain tissue is covered by ependyma (Figure 2–5). These ependymal cells are epithelial cells that have different forms depending on the region in which they are found. In some regions, the epithelial cells of the ependyma have cilia in contact with the CSF (Page et al., 1979). Cilia lining the brain ventricles are morphologically similar to those in the trachea. There are differences in the frequency of beating in different parts of the ventricular system, and the cilia are unable to move particles as they do in the trachea (Roth et al., 1985). Although brain cilia do not seem to move fluid through the system by their beating motion, they may stir the surface molecules to reduce the unstirred layer and increase transport (Nelson and Wright, 1974).

In the region of the floor of the third ventricle, called the median eminence or infundibulum, specialized cells called "tanycytes" connect the hypothalamic nuclei with the ventricular surface. On electron micrographs, tanycytes appear to extend through to the surface of the ependyma. The ventricular surface of the tanycytes has microvilli rather than cilia. The tanycytes are connected by tight junctions that form a diffusion barrier at the ependyma that restricts movement of molecules from CSF to median eminence structures. As the tanycyte processes pass through the median eminence, they end on capillaries. Blebs are seen on the tanycyte surface by scanning electron microscopy that suggest a secretory function. Another possible function

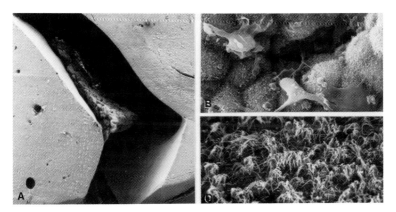

Figure 2–5. A. Scanning electron micrograph of the ventricular system of the adult cat. B. Choroid plexus with microvilli. C. Third ventricle with cilia. (Courtesy of Dr. L. Saland)

is as a conduit for hormones to be transported from the CSF to hypothalamic nuclei, or vice versa, but the anatomy of tight junctions is more suggestive of a barrier function (Martin and Reichlin, 1987).

The anterior region of the third ventricle contains the circumventricular organs, including the median eminence, organum vasculorum of the lamina terminalis, subfornical organ, subcommissural organ, neural lobe, pineal gland, and area postrema. Interestingly, the blood–brain barrier is lacking here, so the hypothalamic cells are exposed to the circulating blood. Nuclei in these areas can act as chemical sensors (Broadwell et al., 1979). The extracellular space of the median eminence is exposed to substances in the blood that can modulate release of the hypothalamic releasing factors. As if to compensate for the absence of the blood–brain barrier, the ependyma over the hypothalamic region of the third ventricle has tight junctions that limit the movement of substances between the hypothalamic nuclei and the CSF. Thus, substances that enter the brain in the hypothalamic region are restricted from moving into the CSF and confined within the brain.

When the ventricles enlarge in hydrocephalus, the ependymal cells are damaged. In the white matter they are flattened and separated from each other so that fluid moves into the white matter. This results in the symptoms of the hydrocephalic syndrome, including gait disturbance, incontinence, and dementia. Frontal white matter fibers are particularly vulnerable to damage.

A layer of pial cells covers the surface of the brain at the outer brain–CSF interface. As found in the ependyma, the pial cells are joined together by gap junctions that allow some substances injected into the CSF to enter the neuropil. Pial adventitia surrounds blood vessels where they penetrate the pial surface (Maynard et al., 1957), whereas the Virchow-Robin space is between the brain cells and the blood vessels (Figure 2–6). Molecules in the CSF penetrate into the neuropil along these spaces.

Rennels et al. (1985) found that injection of HRP into CSF in cats resulted in a rapid filling of the perivascular channels by the protein in both superficial and deep brain regions. These studies suggest that the perivascular pathways are continuous with the subarachnoid space and may be important in the exchange of fluid and molecules between the CSF and ISF. However, the direction of the ISF flow and its magnitude cannot be determined from anatomical studies alone (Figure 2–7).

A different view of the relationship of the subarachnoid space to the perivascular space has emerged from electron and scanning microscopic studies in humans by Hutchings and Weller (1986). In autopsy material from normal subjects, instead of a layer of pial cells accompanying the invaginating cortical blood vessel, they found a continuous sheet of pial cells that separated the CSF in the subarachnoid space from the ISF in the perivascular and subpial space (Figure 2–8). Normally, the pia mater is attached to the basement membrane of the outer glial layer, the glial limitans, of the cortical surface. Similarly, the perivascular glial basement membrane closely adheres to the walls of the vessels. Collagen fibers fill the perivascular com-

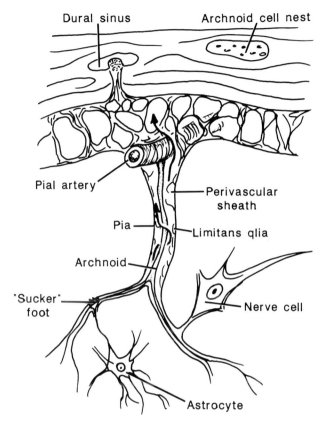

Figure 2–6. Leptomeninges shown with pia–glia surface. An artery is shown penetrating into the cortex. Virchow-Robin perivascular spaces penetrate the cortex along pial vessels. (From Cushing, 1925, after Weed)

partment. The differences between the animal studies and those in humans may be that the pia mater is more substantial in humans than in animals, where it is a thin sheet of cells.

2.4 BLOOD–CSF INTERFACE

Budding from the ependymal surface, the highly vascular choroid plexuses float in the CSF (Figure 2–9). The blood vessels within the plexuses are fenestrated and allow protein to move into the adjacent stroma in a similar manner to the movement of protein in systemic capillaries. Substances from the blood have access to the stroma of the choroid plexus but are prevented from entering the CSF by the tight junctions of the epithelial cells. The apical tight junctions, therefore, form a barrier for the movement of substances from the blood to the CSF.

Histological studies show that Na^+, K^+-ATPase is on the apical surface

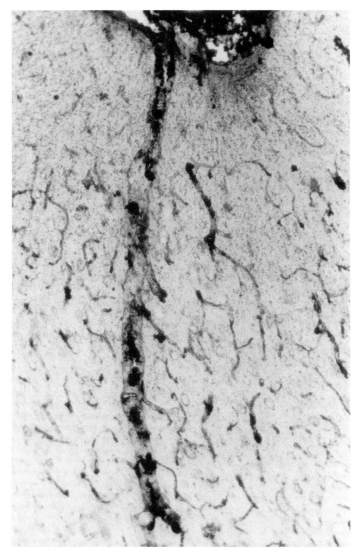

Figure 2–7. Blood vessel surrounded by horseradish peroxidase reaction product 4 hours after intracisternal injection of horseradish peroxidase into the cerebral ventricles in cat. (Original magnification ×40)

of epithelial cells, and magnesium-dependent ATPase is located on the basal membrane (Masuzawa and Sato, 1983). The basal surface of these cells has regions that stain for cyclic nucleotide, suggesting that cyclic AMP (cAMP) may be involved in the secretory process. Other enzymes are found in the epithelial cells of the choroid plexus and probably are involved also in formation of CSF. Carbonic anhydrase and alkaline phosphatase are within the cell.

The surfaces of the choroid plexuses are covered with microvilli. Clefts

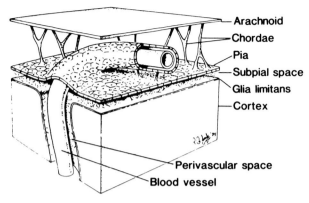

Figure 2–8. Diagramatic representation of the relationship between the subarachnoid and perivascular spaces in humans. The continuity of the perivascular and subpial spaces is seen. (From Hutchings and Weller, 1986)

between cells are seen to extend from the basal surface up to the apical tight junctions. Histologically, the choroid plexuses are similar to other secretory epithelial. The fully developed choroid plexus cell has numerous mitochondria, a Golgi complex, endoplasmic reticulum, and small vesicles (Tennyson and Pappas, 1968). Occasional cilia protrude from between the microvilli on the surface, which may expand the secretory components.

The final site where the blood and the CSF meet is at the arachnoid villi. As at other interfaces, the arachnoid cells covering the brain's surface are joined by tight junctions (Nabeshima et al., 1975) (Figure 2–10). Over the sagittal sinus, the arachnoid cells form villi that protrude into the dural sinuses. Electron microscopy of the arachnoid villi suggests that there are continuous channels through them (Tripathi and Tripathi, 1974). An important function of the arachnoid villi is to prevent blood from the venous sinus from entering the CSF. This is accomplished by the valve-like channels that collapse when pressure is applied from the blood side and open when the CSF pressure increases. Even when the sinus pressure exceeds that in the CSF, there is no reversal of flow. Thus, the arachnoid villi act as one-way valves that open with pressure to allow CSF to drain into the sinuses and close when sinus pressure exceeds that in the CSF to prevent backward flow of blood. An unresolved issue is whether these are actual channels or merely a series of vesicles that can coalesce to form a pseudochannel. Arachnoid cells with the capacity to drain into veins have been found along the spinal cord at the interface of the arachnoid with the spinal roots (Welch and Pollay, 1963).

Electron microscopic studies of the arachnoid reveal a multilayered structure in humans (Alcolado et al., 1988). Five or six layers of cells form the subdural mesothelium. Directly below this layer is the central portion formed from closely opposed, polygonal cells joined by desmosomes and tight junctions; this is the barrier layer. The inner layers are more loosely packed cells that are separated by bundles of collagen fibers. Finally, a very thin layer

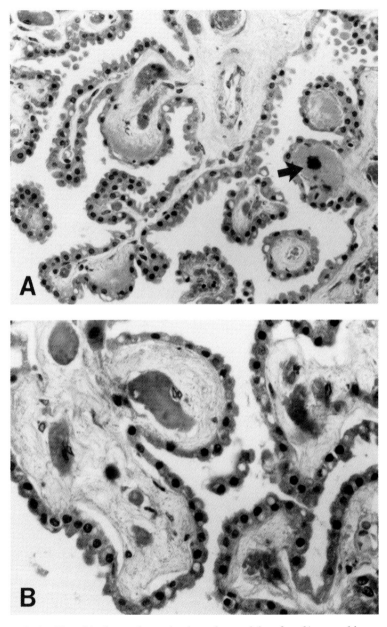

Figure 2–9. Choroid plexus from the lateral ventricle of a 61-year-old woman. Ramifying villous processes consist of connective tissue cores covered by a single layer of cuboidal epithelium. The cores carry blood vessels and contain a rare calcareous deposit (arrow). The epithelium is frequently vacuolated (hematoxylin and eosin; Original magnifications: A, × 294; B, × 460) (Courtesy of Dr. M. Kornfeld).

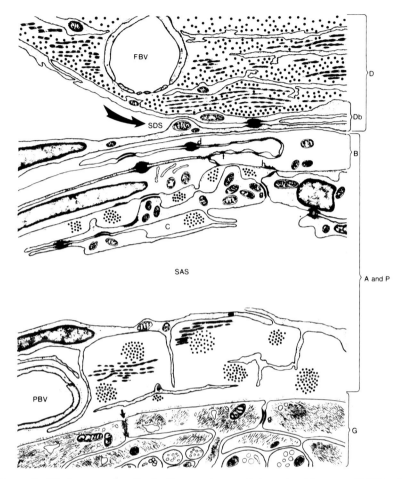

Figure 2–10. Layers of cells in the meninges. Subarachnoid space (SAS) with arachnoid cells and arachnoid barrier layer (B). Tight junctions (t), desmosomes (d), hemidesmosomes (h), and gap junctions (g) are shown. Glia (G), dura (D), fenestrated blood vessels (FBV), subdural space (SDS), and pial blood vessel (PBV) are indicated. (From Nabeshima et al., 1975)

of leptomeningeal cells is found. Traversing the subarachnoid space are sheets of trabeculae that are formed from collagen fibers and contain small blood vessels. The collagen bundles of the trabeculae are continuous with those in the subpial space.

A mechanism of ISF drainage that incorporates movement through the trabeculae traversing the subarachnoid space has been proposed (Krisch et al., 1984). Tracers injected into the brains of rats appeared in the perivascular spaces and the trabeculae, suggesting that ISF drained along the perivascular spaces, into the trabeculae, and out of the brain. To be able to assess their relevance in humans, these findings in the rat need to be repeated in other mammals.

2.5 BLOOD–BRAIN INTERFACE

Endothelial cells are the most important structures that maintain the neuronal environment because of their large surface area as compared to the other interfaces. The capillaries are formed by a single layer of endothelial cells surrounded by a basal lamina. Astrocytic foot processes abut on the capillary walls. Brain capillaries differ from systemic capillaries in that they have tight junctions between the cells, creating a sheet of epithelial cells that limit movement of charged, nonlipid-soluble molecules. These endothelial cells also have an increased number of mitochondria associated with transport systems that deliver essential nutrients, glucose, and amino acids to the brain.

The abluminal surface of the capillary has a Na^+, K^+-ATPase. Other enzymes are located in the endothelial plasma membrane, which performs both a barrier function by metabolizing substances in the blood before they enter brain and a metabolic function by preserving the cell and surrounding nerve cells.

The anatomical basis for the blood–brain barrier is the tight junctions between cerebral capillaries. The original studies of Paul Ehrlich in 1885 showed the existence of the barrier when brain tissue remained unstained after he injected dyes intravenously. However, the precise localization of the barrier occurred when Reese and Karnovsky (1967) demonstrated that intravenously injected HRP was unable to pass the endothelial tight junctions in brain capillaries. Smaller molecules, including microperioxidase and lanthanum ion, also are prevented from passing the barrier (Bundgaard, 1982).

Ultrastructural studies have shown that very few pinocytotic vesicles are present in brain capillaries as compared to systemic ones. However, an increase in pinocytotic vesicles is seen in certain pathological processes, such as increased intracranial pressure and hypertension (Hansson and Johansson, 1980). The increased number of vesicles could represent enhanced transport across the capillary or be a sign of an injured vessel that is losing its capacity to transport substances.

Brain capillaries contain an increased number of mitochondria as compared to systemic capillaries, probably to meet the increased metabolic demand (Oldendorf et al., 1977). An incomplete basement membrane surrounds the endothelial cell. The basement membrane of the cerebral capillary is a basal lamina composed of proteoglycans, laminin, and type IV collagen fibers. It lacks, however, a larger collagen-containing outer layer as is seen in basement membranes in other organs (Sapsford et al., 1983; McArdle et al., 1984). The brain has basal lamina in various other locations: below the ependymal and pial cells, between blood vessels and glial cells, and around astrocytes in contact with connective tissue. In other organs, the basement membrane plays a structural role and is important in filtration. Basement membrane in glomerulus of the kidney is important in filtration of molecules according to charge and size. Vracko (1974) proposed that the basal lamina provides a structural role for the organization of parenchymal and connective tissue elements. Cellular adhension molecules are localized to the interface between astrocytes and blood vessels (Sapsford et al., 1983). Laminin is the main adhesion molecule in brain basal laminas.

Basement membranes are found in regions where substances are exchanged, such as the basal surface of the intestine, the glomerulus of the kidney, and muscle cells (Leonhardt and Desaga, 1975). In other tissues, the basement membranes also are composed of collagen type IV, heparan sulfate, and laminin. The glycoproteins give it a negative charge. In kidney, the glycosaminoglycan matrix of the basement membrane participates in its filtration function by preventing loss of large molecules, and the anions in the membrane allow cations and uncharged molecules to pass more readily through the membrane. Brain basal lamina also appear to have an anionic charge, which is speculated to participate in the function of the blood–brain–barrier (Vorbrodt, 1987).

The basal lamina of brain capillaries is a continuation of the perivascular cell layers around the larger vessels in the Virchow-Robin space. Horseradish peroxidase injected into the CSF of cats filled the Virchow-Robin spaces in a short time and localized to the basal lamina around the capillaries (Rennels et al., 1985). Thus, it is possible that the basal lamina in brain aids in transport of substances.

2.6 EXTRACELLULAR MATRIX

Fifteen to twenty percent of brain tissue is extracellular space, which measures 15–20 nm in width. In other organs, the cells are embedded in a connective tissue matrix that contains collagen fibers. However, extracellular matrix of the brain has very little collagen, and the neurons are embedded in a matrix of glial cells. Earlier investigators thought that the glial cells formed a continuous matrix; *glia* is Greek, meaning "glue." Better definition of the glial cell membranes has shown the presence of a space, which, it has been suggested, contains the complex carbohydrates, such as the glycosaminoglycans, heparan sulfate, chondroitin sulfate, dermatan sulfate, and hyaluronic acid (Margolis et al., 1986).

Although all of the glycosaminoglycans have been found in varying concentrations in developing and mature brain, their exact location in the extracellular space is problematic. The stains ruthenium red and alcian blue, which bind to acidic structures, have been localized in the extracellular space, but the substances to which they are binding remain unknown.

Normal development of brain tissues depends on the extracellular molecules, which provide a substrate for the migration of developing cells from one brain site to another. Cytotactin is an extracellular matrix protein involved in neuron–glial adhesion (Hoffman and Edelman, 1987). It is hydrolyzed by chondroitinase, suggesting that it has chondroitin sulfate proteoglycan.

Extracellular matrix molecules have an important role in the developing brain, where they determine the migration patterns of newly formed cells,

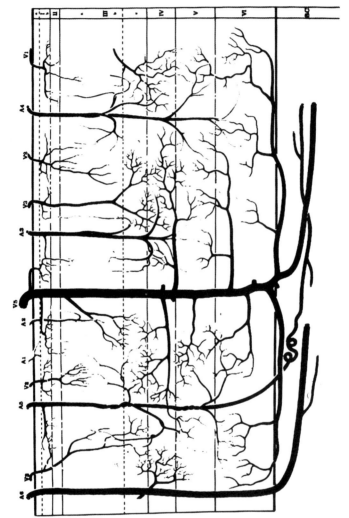

Figure 2–11. Drawing of the morphological features of intracortical arteries and veins. Arteries are divided into six groups (A1–A6) and veins into five, (V1–V5). I, II, III, IV, V, VI, cortical cellular layers; SC, subcortical white matter. (From Duvernoy et al., 1981)

but the role of matrix molecules in the mature brain is less well understood. One possible role of cell surface molecules is in tumor recognition. Glioma cells from human brain tumors grown in culture have a glycosaminoglycan coat that prevents them from being destroyed by cytotoxic lymphocytes. This coat appears to contain hyaluronic acid, since application of hyaluronidase to the culture allows the lymphocytes to destroy the tumor (Oberc-Greenwood et al., 1986).

2.7 BRAIN VASCULATURE

All blood flowing to the human brain comes from either the carotid or the vertebral arteries. Anastomotic channels between the carotid or anterior circulation and the vertebrobasilar or posterior circulation occur primarily at the circle of Willis and, to a lesser extent, over the surface of the brain in the leptomeningeal arteries. The lack of extensive anastomoses between arterial territories results in cerebral ischemia when vessels are occluded, as in stroke.

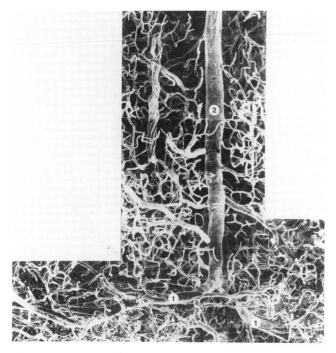

Figure 2–12. Intracortical vein. 1, subcortical and deep branches; 2, trunk of the vein. (From Duvernoy et al., 1981)

The arteries develop on the surface of the brain and penetrate into the deep structures. Scharrer (1940) used selective injection of arteries and veins to show that there are no anastomotic channels between the arteries and veins on the surface of the brain. The brain blood vessels are end-arteries, the occlusion of which results in a stroke. Scharrer studied the evolution of vascular patterns and found that the marsupials (opossums) have a loop sys-

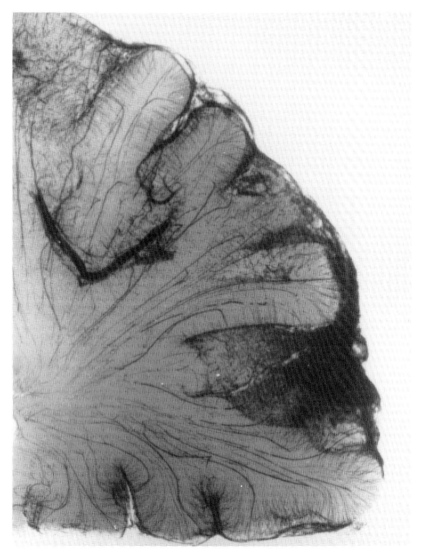

Figure 2–13. Soft x-ray picture of brain injected with radiopaque material after death in a 51-year-old female showing arterial branches of the cerebral cortex and white matter. The radial pattern of cortical, subcortical, and medullary arteries toward the lateral ventricle are seen. (From Akima et al., 1986)

tem in which the arteries fold back onto the veins so that each artery enters the cortex with a vein. The Placentalia (e.g., monkey, cat, rabbit), on the other hand, have a network-like vascular pattern with the arteries entering the cortical surface at one point, forming capillaries, and exiting as veins at another point.

Blood vessels penetrate into the cortex from the pia perpendicular to the surface. The density of the cortical vasculature corresponds to the cellular density of the cortex. Arteries penetrate the superficial layers and branch at the middle layers or course through the cortex into the white matter (Figure 2–11). At the gray–white junction, they turn at a 90° angle to follow the fiber tracts of the cortex (Duvernoy et al., 1981). There is a correlation between vascular density and increased cellularity in the cortical layers. The densest vascularity occurs in the highly cellular layers III, IV, and V. The vascular cortex turns into a poorly vascular subcortical white matter. The vessels in the white matter follow the fiber tracts and turn around the cortical sulci. Reconstruction of a large cortical vein from scanning electron micrographs of human autopsy material perfused with plastic embedding materials and with the tissue dissolved away is shown in Figure 2–12.

Human brains perfused after death with barium and x-rayed in sections (microangiography) showed that arteries course from the cortex toward the ventricle (Figure 2–13). Scanning electron micrographs of aging brains showed that small arterial branches intertwine in rope-like structures that correlate with the extent of atrophy (Akima et al., 1986). The intertwining arterial rami were formed from proximal to distal ends and always in a clockwise direction. Occasionally, a looping artery, as in a glomerular loop formation, was seen at the cortical–subcortical junction. Twisted vessels could interfere either with tissue perfusion or with perivascular transport.

REFERENCES

Akima, M., Nonaka, H., Kagesaura, M., Tanaka, K.: A study of the microvasculature of the cerebral cortex: Fundamental architecture and its senile change in the frontal cortex. Lab. Invest. 55:482–489, 1986.

Alcolado, R., Weller, R. O., Parrish, E. P., Garrod, D.: The cranial arachnoid and pia mater in man: Anatomical and ultrastructural observations. Neuropathol. Appl. Neurobiol. 14:1–17, 1988.

Brightman, M. W., Reese, T. S.: Junctions between intimately apposed cell membranes in the vertebrate brain. J. Cell. Biol. 40:648–677, 1969.

Broadwell, R. D., Oliver, C., Brightman, M. W.: Localization of neurophysin within organelles associated with protein synthesis and packaging in the hypothalamoneurohypophysial system: An immunocytochemical study. Proc. Natl. Acad. Sci. USA 76:5999–6003, 1979.

Bundgaard, M.: Ultrastructure of frog cerebral and pial microvessels and their impermeability to lanthanum ions. Brain Res. 241:57–65, 1982.

Carpenter, M. B., Sutin, J.: Human Neuroanatomy. Baltimore: Williams & Wilkins, 1983.

Cushing, H.: The Third Circulation. Oxford: Oxford University Press, 1925.

Duvernoy, H. M., Delon, S., Vannson, J. L.: Cortical blood vessels of the human
    brain. Brain Res. Bull. 7:519–579, 1981.

Gabriel, R. S.: *Textbook of Child Neurology*. Menkes, J. H., ed. Philadelphia: Lea
    & Febiger, 1974:130–140.

Hansson, H. A., Johansson, B. B.: Induction of pinocytosis in cerebral vessels by
    acute hypertension and by hyperosmolar solutions. J. Neurosci. Res. 5:183–
    190, 1980.

Hoffman, S., Edelman, G. M.: A proteoglycan with HNK-1 antigenic determinants
    is a neuron-associated ligand for cytotactin. Proc. Natl. Acad. Sci. USA
    84:2523–2527, 1987.

Hutchings, M., Weller, R. O.: Anatomical relationships of the pia mater to cerebral
    blood vessels in man. J. Neurosurg. 65:316–325, 1986.

Krisch, B., Leonhardt, H., Oksche, A.: Compartments and perivascular arrange-
    ment of the meninges covering the cerebral cortex of the rat. Cell Tissue Res.
    238:459–474, 1984.

Langman, J., Guerrant, R. L., Freeman, B. G.: Behavior of neuroepithelial cells
    during closure of the neural tube. J. Comp. Neurol. 127:399–411, 1966.

Leonhardt, H., Desaga, U.: Recent observations on ependyma and subependymal
    basement membrane. Acta. Neurochir. 31:153–159, 1975.

Margolis, R. U., Aquino, D. A., Klinger, M. M., Ripellino, J. A., Margolis, R. K.:
    Structure and localization of nervous tissue proteoglycans. Ann. NY Acad.
    Sci. 481:46–54, 1986.

Martin, J. B., Reichlin, S.: *Clinical Neuroendocrinology*. Philadelphia: FA Davis
    Co., 1987:22–24.

Masuzawa, T., Sato, F.: The enzyme histochemistry of the choroid plexus. Brain
    106:55–99, 1983.

Maynard, E. A., Schultz, R. L., Pease, D. C.: Electron microscopy of the vascular
    bed of rat cerebral cortex. Am. J. Anat. 100:409–434, 1957.

McArdle, J. P., Muller, H. K., Roff, B. T., Murphy, W. H.: Basal lamina rede-
    velopment in tumors metastatic to brain: An immunoperoxidase study using
    an antibody to type IV collagen. Int. J. Cancer 34:633–638, 1984.

Millen, J. N., Wollam, D. H. M.: *The Anatomy of Cerebrospinal Fluid*. Oxford:
    Oxford University Press, 1962.

Nabeshima, S., Reese, T. S., Landis, D. M., Brightman, M. W.: Junctions in the
    meninges and marginal glia. J. Comp. Neurol. 164:127–169, 1975.

Nelson, D. J., Wright, E. M.: The distribution, activity and function of the cilia in
    the frog brain. J. Physiol. (Lond) 243:63–78, 1974.

Oberc-Greenwood, M. A., Muul, L. M., Gately, M. K., Kornblith, P. L., Smith,
    B. H.: Ultrastructural features of the lymphocyte-stimulated halos produced
    by human glioma-derived cells in vitro. J. Neurooncol. 3:387–396, 1986.

Oldendorf, W. H., Cornford, M. E., Brown, W. J.: The large apparent work ca-
    pability of the blood–brain barrier: A study of the mitochondrial content of
    capillary endothelial cells in brain and other tissues of the rat. Ann. Neurol.
    1:409–417, 1977.

Page, R. B., Rosenstein, J. M., Leure-duPree, A. E.: The morphology of extra-
    choroidal ependyma overlying gray and white matter in the rabbit lateral ven-
    tricle. Anat. Rec. 194:67–81, 1979.

Reese, T. S., Karnovsky, M. J.: Fine structural localization of a blood–brain barrier
    to exogenous peroxidase. J. Cell. Biol. 34:207–217, 1967.

Rennels, M. L., Gregory, T. F., Blaumanis, O. R., Fujimoto, K., Grady, P. A.:

Evidence for a "paravascular" fluid circulation in the mammalian central nervous system, provided by the rapid distribution of tracer protein throughout the brain from the subarachnoid space. Brain Res. 326:47–63, 1985.

Roth, Y., Kimbi, Y., Edery, H., Ahorouson, E., Priel, Z.: Ciliary motility in brain ventricular system and trachea of hamsters. Brain Res. 330:291–297, 1985.

Sapsford, I., Buontempo, J., Weller, R. O.: Basement membrane surfaces and perivascular compartments in normal human brain and glial tumors. A scanning electron microscopic study. Neuropathol. Appl. Neurobiol. 9:181–194, 1983.

Schade, J. P., Ford, D. H.: *Basic Neurology.* Amsterdam: Elsevier Publishing Co., 1965.

Scharrer, E.: Arteries and veins in the mammalian brain. Anat. Rec. 78:173–196, 1940.

Stewart, P. A., Wiley, M. J.: Developing nervous tissue induces formation of blood–brain barrier characteristics in invading endothelial cells: A study using quail chick transplantation chimeras. Dev. Biol. 84:183–192, 1981.

Tennyson, V. M., Pappas, G. D.: The fine structure of the choroid plexus: Adult and developmental stages. Prog. Brain Res. 29:63–85, 1968.

Tripathi, B. J., Tripathi, R. C.: Vacuolar transcellular channels as a drainage pathway for cerebrospinal fluid. J. Physiol. (Lond) 239:195–206, 1974.

Vorbrodt, A. W.: Demonstration of anionic sites on the luminal and abluminal fronts of endothelial cells with poly-1-lysine-gold complex. J. Histol. Cytol. 35:1261–1266, 1987.

Vracko, R.: Basal lamina scaffold, anatomy and significance for maintenance of orderly tissue structure. Am. J. Pathol. 77:314–346, 1974.

Welch, K., Pollay, M.: The spinal arachnoid villi of the monkeys *Cercopithecus aethiops sabaeus* and *Macaca irus.* Anat. Rec. 145:43–48, 1963.

3

Physiology of Cerebrospinal and Interstitial Fluids

3.1 INTRODUCTION

Normal CSF is clear and colorless, with a low protein content and few cells. The CSF is secreted by the choroid plexuses and extrachoroidally by the capillaries and cellular metabolism. The human nervous system contains an estimated 120 ml of CSF, of which 20 ml is within the ventricles. Since about 500 ml of CSF is produced daily in humans, steady drainage is essential to avoid excess accumulation and increased pressure. Drainage of CSF occurs primarily across the arachnoid villi and into the lymphatics.

Until recently, the function of the CSF was assumed to be to buffer the brain against trauma (McComb, 1983). Although the CSF does cushion the impact on the brain of a blow to the head, a more important role of CSF is to act as a lymph system for the brain (Weed, 1914, 1935). The brain lacks an actual lymphatic network, but the ISF provides an intracerebral transport system that allows movement of nutrients, toxins, and products of metabolism. Transport within brain tissue occurs between cells in the extracellular space and along the perivascular spaces.

The CSF and ISF are in contact across the brain surfaces, and gap junctions between the ependymal and pial cells allow the exchange of molecules between CSF and ISF (Brightman and Reese, 1969). Direct continuity of the CSF and ISF allows substances in one compartment to be transferred to the other. For example, injection of drugs into the CSF by lumbar puncture bypasses the blood–brain barrier and allows the injected substance to enter the brain. Similarly, substances formed in the brain appear in the CSF; thus, the CSF reflects brain metabolic activity. Since the concentration of the substance in the CSF is generally lower than its level in the brain, the CSF acts as a sink, with the substance moving down a concentration gradient (Davson, 1967). In response to pathological conditions, the CSF accumulates abnormal amounts of the metabolites of neurotransmitters, neuropeptides, and abnormal proteins.

3.2 FORMATION, CIRCULATION, AND ABSORPTION OF CSF

Choroid plexuses in the lateral, third, and fourth ventricles secrete the major portion of the CSF and participate in the regulation of the ionic composition of the CSF. Formation of CSF could potentially occur by two mechanisms: filtration of fluid across the choroid plexus epithelial cells or active secretion of fluid by ionic mechanisms. For many years it was thought that filtration was the primary mechanism for CSF formation. This view was changed when Ames et al. (1964) developed methods for collecting the freshly formed CSF in animals by filling the ventricles with oil and trapping the newly secreted CSF for measurements of ion content. In a series of elegant experiments, they were able to show that the CSF regulates the content of potassium and sodium. Since the ionic content of CSF differed from that expected for an ultrafiltrate of plasma, the fluid was formed by an active secretory process that kept potassium levels in CSF within a very narrow range and allowed sodium content to fluctuate with serum levels.

Na^+, K^+-ATPase and carbonic anhydrase are the major enzymes that control CSF secretion. Inhibition of these enzymes by ouabain and acetazolamide, respectively, reduces CSF formation. Histochemical studies show that the Na^+, K^+-ATPase is located on the microvilli of the apical (CSF facing) surface of the epithelial cells of the choroid plexus and that carbonic anhydrase is within the cells (Masuzawa and Sato, 1983). Cyclic nucleotides appear to be involved in CSF secretion. Injection of cholera toxin into the ventricle, which stimulates adenylate cyclase, increases the CSF formation rate (Epstein et al., 1977). Adenylate cyclase is located along the basal plasmalemma of the choroid plexus (Masuzawa and Sato, 1983). Recently, a neuropeptide was shown to affect the rate of CSF formation. Atrial natriuretic factor (ANF) is released by the heart atria in response to water overload. When ANF was infused into the CSF, it reduced the CSF formation rate (Steardo and Nathanson, 1987).

Although the choroid plexus and the ependymal cells lining the ventricles have a common epithelial cell origin, they differ in their secretory properties and enzymatic make-up. The ATPase located on the apical surface of the choroid plexus appears on the basal (brain facing) surface of the ventricular epithelium. Furthermore, the adenylate cyclase is found on the apical rather than the basal surface of the ependymal cells. The reason for the reorientation of epithelial cells within the ventricle is unknown. Perhaps the blood vessels that form the choroid plexus stimulate the enzyme orientation and tight junction formation in the overlying epithelial cells. Nevertheless, the enzymatic reorientation may be important in fluid regulation by neuropeptide-sensitive ependymal cells (Rosenberg et al., 1986).

The mechanism of CSF secretion in mammals is shown schematically in Figure 3–1. Fenestrated capillaries allow fluid, protein, and electrolytes to escape into the stroma underlying the epithelial cells of the choroid plexus, since the barrier is formed by tight junctions at the epithelial cell apical surface rather than at the capillaries. Sodium enters the epithelial cell in exchange for hydrogen. Sodium is removed from the cell by an exchange at the apical surface of three intracellular sodium ions for two potassium ions in the CSF. The extra ion pumped by ATPase into the CSF increases the osmotic pressure on the surface, which results in the formation of CSF. Sodium ions accumulate on the apical surface as a result of the imbalance in their exchange with potassium. Excess sodium increases the osmolality at the CSF surface of the choroid cell. Water is removed from the cell by the osmotic pressure.

Pollay (1975) proposed that CSF was formed by a standing gradient cre-

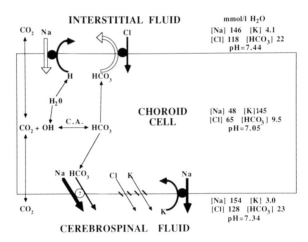

Figure 3–1. Model for ion transporters and channels in the mammalian choroidal epithelium. Primary active Na-K pumping on the apical (CSF facing) membrane lowers the cell [Na], thereby providing the driving force for the parallel operation of the secondary active antiporters, Na-H and Cl-HCO_3, on the basolateral surface. The abundance of H_2O and CO_2 from catabolism furnishes substrate for the carbonic anhydrase (C.A.)-catalyzed generation of HCO_3. K, Cl, and HCO_3 leave the cell by electrochemically downhill movement via conductance pathways. NaHCO_3 symport has been hypothesized. The ion concentrations and pH values for the three compartments (blood, choroid plexus, CSF) are baseline values in ketamine-anesthetized animals. Cell values were averaged for lateral ventricle choroid plexus and fourth ventricle choroid plexus. CSF secretion essentially is net movement of NaCl and NaHCO_3 across the barrier into the ventricles. Filled and unfilled arrows designate active and nonactive transport, respectively. Curved arrows represent potential for the transported ion to be recycled, for example, cellular HCO_3 extruded into ISF can be converted to CO_2 for diffusive uptake by the cell, or actively accumulated K can backdiffuse into the CSF. The interior of the cell is approximately 45 mV negative to both ISF and CSF. (Courtesy of Dr. C. Johanson, Brown University)

ated in the lateral clefts of the cells by sodium transport analogous to the situation in the gallbladder. The sodium accumulated in these clefts, with water following along an increasing osmotic gradient. Although the exact mechanism of CSF formation remains to be resolved, it is well accepted that an excess of ATPase molecules found on the apical end of the cleft creates an osmotic gradient with an excess of sodium ions on the apical surface.

As part of the CSF formation, HCO_3^- and Cl^- are exchanged between the CSF and plasma. Bicarbonate plays an important role in CSF formation by carbonic anhydrase. To balance the movement of HCO_3^-, there is a Cl^--HCO_3^- exchange that is driven by the need to maintain a steady-state intracellular HCO_3^- level (Johanson et al., 1985).

Although the primary driving force for CSF formation in the frog is Na^+-K^+ exchange at the apical surface, the HCO_3^- ion is linked to CSF secretion by AMP (Saito and Wright, 1983). Cholera toxin is a potent stimulus of AMP, and it causes an increase in CSF formation (Epstein et al., 1977). The mechanism appears to be related to an increase in HCO_3^- transport. There are α-adrenergic receptors associated with adenylate cyclase in the choroid plexuses (Nathanson, 1980). Lindvall and Owman (1981) have shown adrenergic, cholinergic, and peptidergic nerve innervations of mammalian choroid plexus and inhibition of CSF secretion by cholinergic and adrenergic agonists.

The rate of CSF formation depends on the weight of the choroid plexus and varies among species (Cserr, 1971). In humans, the rate is 0.35 ml/minute, whereas in rabbit, the rate is 0.01 ml/minute. However, formation of CSF as a function of choroid plexus weight is remarkably constant over a range of species (Table 3–1). Although several drugs can inhibit CSF production for a short period, they have proven to be of limited clinical use because of either their time frame of action or their toxicity. Acetazolamide, an inhibitor of carbonic anhydrase, reduces the CSF formation rate by up to 40 percent. Inhibitors of ATPase, such as digitalis, also reduce CSF formation; but the effect is too short-lived to be of clinical importance. Increased CSF pressure reduces CSF formation only slightly (Heisey et al., 1962).

Table 3–2 lists factors that influence the rate of CSF formation. Hyperosmolality produced by intravenous mannitol reduces CSF production by 50 percent (Sahar et al., 1978; Rosenberg et al., 1980), and this drug is used clinically in patients with raised intracranial pressure to lower the pres-

Table 3–1.   Rate of CSF Formation in Various Species

Species	μl/minute	μl/minute/mg Choroid Plexus
Rabbit	10	0.43
Cat	20	0.5
Dog	50	0.63
Goat	154	0.36
Human	350	0.18

From Cserr, 1971.

Table 3–2. Factors That Influence CSF Formation

	Substance	Site of Action
Increase production	Cholera toxin	Adenylate cyclase
	Adrenergic stimulation	Adenylate cyclase
Decrease production	Oubain	Na^+, K^+-ATPase
	Acetazolamide	Carbonic anhydrase
	Hyperosmolality	Choroid plexus capillaries
	Hypothermia	Decreased metabolism
	Atrial natriuretic hormone	Cyclic GMP

sure temporarily (Wise and Chater, 1962). Hypothermia influences CSF production by reducing cerebral metabolism.

Circulation of CSF begins in the cerebral ventricles, with the fluid exiting through the foramina of Luschka and Magendie into the cisterna magna. Flow of CSF within the subarachnoid space can follow two patterns (Figure 3–2). It can move up over the convexities to be absorbed into the blood across the arachnoid villi, or it can mix with the CSF in the spinal sac for subsequent removal into the vascular structures around the spinal cord or transport up over the hemispheres.

The flow of CSF can be determined clinically by the use of radioisotope cisternography, which is the injection of radioactive substances into the lumbar spinal fluid (DiChiro et al., 1964). Cisternography is done with the gamma emitter technetium labeled to diethylenetriaminepentaacetic acid (DTPA), a large chelating agent. After injection of the isotope into the lumbar sac, nuclear brain scans are done at 2, 24, and 48 hours. The radioactive substances are transported slowly toward the head. If the molecular weight is high, the molecules remain within the CSF in the subarachnoid space and are reabsorbed at the arachnoid villi. Lower molecular weight substances diffuse from the spinal canal through the vascular plexuses surrounding the cord (DiChiro et al., 1976). Normally, substances injected into the lumbar sac remain outside the ventricles. When they enter the ventricular system, it is a sign of brain atrophy or communicating hydrocephalus. If the injected substance not only enters the ventricles but also remains within the ventricles for 48 hours or longer, it may indicate transependymal absorption of CSF. Since fluid moves from the brain into the CSF (extrachoroidal production) and out into the subarachnoid space through the foramina of Luschka and Magendie, the reverse of this normal pattern, as CSF moves back into the brain across the ependyma, indicates a pathological flow pattern. With time, the transependymal flow interferes with periventricular cellular function and permanently damages the tissue.

The absorption of CSF at the arachnoid villi is pressure sensitive (Figure 3–3). As the CSF pressure increases, so does the amount of CSF absorbed. Several explanations have been offered to describe the absorption process. It has been proposed that the arachnoid villi act as valves that open with raised pressure and close as the pressure falls (Welch and Friedman, 1960). However, the basis for this mechanism is controversial, and some investi-

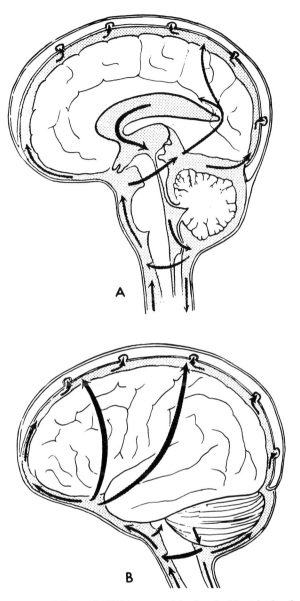

Figure 3–2. Patterns of flow of CSF in normal brain. A. Ventricular formation of CSF with exits at the foramina of Luschka and Magendie. B. Flow around the spinal cord or up over the convexity. (From Milhorat, 1972)

gators have suggested that channels through the arachnoid appear and coalesce as the pressure is increased (Tripathi and Tripathi, 1974). Particles of larger size may be trapped by the arachnoid in the channels. Red blood cells released by subarachnoid hemorrhage, for example, are trapped in the arachnoid villi and impair CSF absorption (Alksne and Lovings, 1972). The

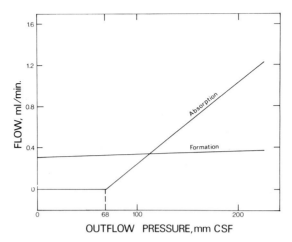

Figure 3–3. Absorption of CSF is pressure dependent, whereas the formation rate is insensitive to pressure. The pressure at which the rate of formation and the rate of absorption intersect is the normal CSF pressure. (Modified from Cutler et al., 1968)

blood cells in the CSF can impair absorption and lead to enlargement of the ventricular system. Transient hydrocephalus after subarachnoid hemorrhage may occur and, at times, requires surgical insertion of a shunt to divert fluid from the ventricles to the pleural or abdominal cavity. Other materials also can interfere with CSF absorption if present in high concentration in the CSF in pathological conditions, for example, white blood cells in meningitis and marked increases in protein in postinfectious polyneuropathy (Guillain-Barré syndrome).

Infusion of artificial CSF into the lumbar sac while the pressure is recorded has been used as a test of the absorptive capacity of the arachnoid villi. Normal individuals can tolerate infusion of CSF at rates twice those of production without an increase in pressure (Katzman and Hussey, 1970). When the CSF absorptive mechanism is impaired, there is a rise in pressure as the fluid is infused (Hussey et al., 1970).

3.3 CSF COMPOSITION

Sodium is the most abundant ion in the CSF, and it is important in transport and osmoregulation. Tracer studies with ^{24}Na have shown that the CSF and plasma levels are closely related (Davson and Pollay, 1963). Acetazolamide, an inhibitor of carbonic anhydrase, slows the entrance of radiolabeled sodium into the CSF (Davson and Luck, 1957). Vasopressin enhances the movement of sodium from blood to brain (Fishman, 1959). The exchange time for ^{24}Na transport from blood to brain is about 2 hours and depends on the region sampled.

Radiolabeled sodium accumulated in periventricular regions after intravenous injection (Smith and Rapoport, 1986). The reason for this is that choroid plexus epithelium is about 300 times more permeable to ^{24}Na than is the cerebrovascular endothelium. Cerebral capillaries have a membrane permeability to sodium of 1.4×10^{-7} cm/second, which is similar to their permeability to mannitol and in the same range as tight-junctioned epithelial membranes (Rapoport, 1976).

The electrical charge across a membrane is determined by the distribution of charged ions. In epithelial membranes, the electrical charge is regulated by the Na^+, K^+-ATPase pump. Tight-junctioned epithelial sheets have a high electrical resistance, whereas those with leaky junctions have a lower resistance (Crone and Christensen, 1981). Thus, measurement of the electrical resistance across the secreting epithelium gives an indication of the tightness of the junctions. The greater permeability of the choroid plexus epithelium is due in part to leaky intercellular junctions with an electrical resistance of 26 ohm/cm^2, which is similar to that of other leaky epithelium. For comparison, the electrical resistance of frog brain capillary is 1,900 ohm/cm^2, and tight epithelium, such as toad bladder, is over 4,000 ohm/ cm^2 (Olesen and Crone, 1986). Choroid plexus epithelium has a lower permeability to potassium than to sodium, and the reverse is true at the capillary (Table 3–3).

Potassium concentration is maintained within a very narrow range in the CSF (Ames et al., 1964). The normal CSF potassium is approximately 3 mEq/liter. Changes in plasma potassium have little effect on the CSF potassium (Bradbury et al., 1963). Even at very high plasma levels, the CSF potassium remains within the normal range (Katzman and Pappius, 1973). Transport across the blood–brain barrier is limited, and the half-time of exchange for potassium is 24 hours. When potassium levels are increased in the CSF, sodium is exchanged for potassium by an active transport mechanism. Ouabain, an inhibitor of ATPase, interferes with the exchange of sodium and potassium. Potassium is critical for neuronal function and effects the release of neurotransmitters. Therefore, it is maintained at a constant level in the extracellular fluid.

Calcium in the CSF normally ranges between 2 and 3 mEq/liter compared to plasma levels of 4–5.5 mEq/liter. Calcium is secreted from the choroid plexus and has a similar value in various CSF spaces. The rate of calcium

Table 3–3. Permeability of Capillary and Choroid Plexus

	Permeability (cm/second)	
Substance	Capillary ($\times 10^7$)	Choroid Plexus
^{42}K	13.5	190
^{22}Na	1.4	380
^{36}Cl	0.93	420
^{14}C-Mannitol	1.5	14

From Smith and Rapoport, 1986.

entry from blood to CSF is relatively independent of the serum calcium. The ratio of CSF to serum calcium in humans is around 0.50 (Woodbury et al., 1968). The low CSF levels of calcium are maintained by transport mechanisms between blood and CSF.

Both acute and chronic changes in plasma calcium have little effect on brain calcium levels. Fluctuations of plasma calcium from 1 to 7 mmol/liter in dogs change CSF calcium from 1 to 2 mmol/liter (Morgulis and Perley, 1930). Similarly, brain calcium remains constant during acute changes (Wong and Bradbury, 1975). Young rats fed diets low or high in calcium showed a 40 percent fall or a 30 percent rise, respectively, in total plasma calcium. Brain levels remained within 10 percent of those in controls (Murphy et al., 1986). Although calcium enters the brain at the various interfaces comprising the blood–brain barrier, transport across the choroid plexus is the dominant route for calcium entry from blood to brain (Tai et al., 1986).

Regulation of calcium is essential for normal brain function. A marked increase in brain calcium produces impairment in thinking and can lead to coma, whereas very low levels of calcium cause seizures (Katzman and Pappius, 1973). In order to maintain calcium homeostasis, active transport of calcium at the blood–brain barrier is necessary. Both the cerebrovascular endothelium and the choroid plexus participate in this process (Murphly et al., 1986).

Extracellular levels of unbound calcium are higher than intracellular levels. Calcium within the cell is sequestered in mitochondria and smooth endoplasmic reticulum. Entry of calcium into the cell occurs either by a change in the voltage across the membrane that accompanies depolarization or by agonist-operated channels activated by excitatory neurotransmitters. During pathological changes, such as anoxia, potassium concentration rises in the extracellular space, and the calcium levels fall (Nicholson et al., 1977). The extracellular calcium enters the cell and leads to a cascade of molecular events that lead to permanent cell damage.

Postsynaptic calcium channels are activated by glutamate and aspartate (Siesjo, 1988). Both amino acids are excitatory neurotransmitters ubiquitously distributed in brain tissue. The excitatory receptors have been found in high concentrations in the hippocampus and other regions sensitive to ischemic–anoxic injury. Glutamate-sensitive channels open a sodium channel that allows sodium and chloride to enter the cell and this channel also permits calcium to pass. The glutamate-receptor channel is antagonized by magnesium, which may be important in the therapeutic action of magnesium (Nowak et al., 1984). Although calcium entry is a normal consequence of cell excitation by glutamate, excess calcium within the cell can lead to the activation of cellular processes that are detrimental to the cell, such as breakdown of cellular membranes and formation of products of inflammation (Rothman and Olney, 1986).

Protein content is normally 20–40 mg/100 ml in the CSF compared to 5–7 gm/100 ml in serum. Choroid plexuses and the cerebral capillaries have tight junctions between cells that restrict movement of protein from blood to brain. Albumin is the main protein in CSF, comprising 50–70 percent of the total CSF proteins, whereas gamma-globulins are normally between 5 and 12 percent of the total CSF protein (Fishman, 1980). When the blood–brain barrier is damaged, protein leaks into the CSF. Since albumin is the protein found in highest concentration in the blood, it enters the CSF in the greatest amount. Other proteins enter in proportion to their concentration in the blood. However, in some illnesses there is a selective increase in gamma-globulins, which are thought to be secreted by white blood cells residing within the nervous system. Generally, inflammatory and demyelinating diseases are associated with the selective increase in gamma-globulins, which may be accompanied by an increase in inflammatory cells.

3.4 INTERSTITIAL FLUID

The composition of the ISF is thought to be similar to that of the CSF because of the continuity of the two fluids across the ependymal and pial surfaces. Formation of ISF is thought to occur by active transport processes at the cerebral capillary (Rapoport, 1976). Cerebral capillaries act as secretory epithelium (Crone, 1986). They have a high density of mitochondria (Oldendorf et al., 1977) and an ATPase pump on the surface facing the brain tissue (Betz and Goldstein, 1978). Estimates of the amount of CSF coming from ISF production range from 30 to 60 percent, depending on the species studied and the method of measurement (Milhorat, 1971) (Figure 3–4).

The brain lacks a lymphatic system for intracerebral transport of substances; instead, transport occurs between cells and along perivascular pathways. Molecular transport between cells is by diffusion with or without bulk flow (Cserr et al., 1974; Rosenberg et al., 1980; Pullen et al., 1987). Diffusion is a passive process dependent on the molecular weight, extracellular matrix, and time. Diffusion is efficient for short distances, and bulk flow is more rapid for greater distances. Bulk flow follows pressure and osmotic gradients (Rosenberg et al., 1978). The importance of bulk flow is that it is capable of moving molecules of high molecular weights from one intracerebral site to another more efficiently than by diffusion alone. Removal of substances of different molecular weights following direct injection occurs by bulk flow away from a site of intracerebral injection (Cserr et al., 1981). This means that molecules of different sizes can be cleared at similar rates. The driving force for bulk flow in the extracellular space is most likely formation of ISF and may be aided by the pulsations of blood vessels (Rennels et al., 1985).

The extracellular matrix in brain is thought to contain complex carbohydrate molecules (Table 3–4). The main extracellular molecules are the glycosaminoglycans: hyaluronic acid, heparan sulfate, dermatan sulfate, and chondroitin sulfate. Hyaluronic acid is highly hygroscopic and is found in larger amounts in the gray matter than in the white matter (Margolis and Margolis, 1977). Newborns have a high hyaluronic acid content in the brain, which is thought to account for the higher water content. The exact nature

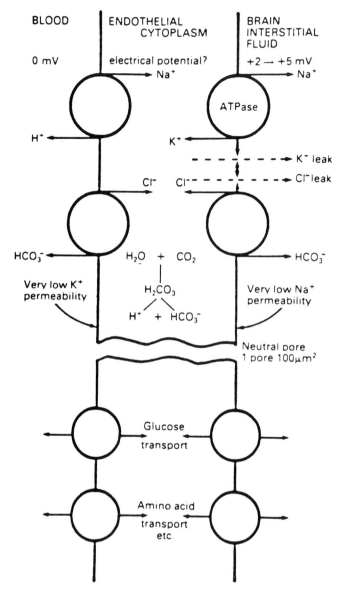

Figure 3–4. Possible transport systems in cerebral endothelium. On the luminal side are a coupled Na-H antiport system and a Cl-HCO3 exchanger. In the abluminal membrane is a coupled Na-K pump driven by energy from ATP hydrolysis, pumping potassium ions out of the interstitium. This membrane also contains a Cl-HCO3 exchanger. The cell chloride (that follows the net Na transport) leaves the cell by electrodiffusion. The junction between two endothelial cells represents the very low conductance passive pathway that is present in all tight epithelial membranes and presumably also in the blood–brain barrier. Only two of the many equilibrating transport systems for organic solutes are indicated, the glucose transporter and the amino acid transporter (of which there are various types). It is suggested that the luminal cell membrane has an extremely low permeability to potassium, whereas the abluminal membrane has a very low Na permeability. (From Crone, 1986)

Table 3–4. Extracellular Matrix Molecules and Possible Functions

Matrix Molecules	Functions of Matrix
Glycoproteins	Bind calcium and electrolytes
Fibronectin	Restrict diffusion of neurotransmitters
Glycosaminoglycans	Exclude toxic substances
Hyaluronic acid	Provide structure
Chondroitin sulfate	Maintain cellular surface receptors
Dermatan sulfate	
Heparan sulfate	

of the extracellular matrix in mature animals, however, is debatable. Light microscopic studies with alcian blue, which stains the acidic extracellular matrix, suggest the presence of hyaluronic acid. Furthermore, injection of hyaluronidase into the CSF enhances the spread of substances through brain tissue and alters electrical impedance (Wang and Adey, 1969). However, antibodies to chondroitin sulfate and probes against hyaluronic acid in the extracellular matrix material have failed to demonstrate the nature of the matrix (Margolis et al., 1986). Probes for the localization of hyaluronic acid in brain tissue showed dense staining in rat brain in presumptive white matter during the first 2 weeks of life but lack of extracellular staining in mature animals. Antibodies to chondroitin sulfate showed an extracellular pattern after birth, with progression to intracellular staining as the animals matured. Thus, the role of glycosaminoglycans in nervous tissue function is unclear. Their high concentration in developing brains suggests that they are important in cell migration through the watery matrix. In mature brains, they may play a role in binding of cations and in osmotic regulation.

Invertebrates have an extracellular matrix material that affects the small ions. In crustaceans, the material in the space is predominantly hyaluronic acid, and the highly charged matrix binds small ions, such as calcium (Lane et al., 1977). Nicholson and Rice (1987) were unable to demonstrate an effect of calcium on diffusion in isolated mammalian tissue, however. During pathological changes, such as hypoxia–ischemia, the extracellular space decreases, and these changes may interfere with normal intracellular transport.

Intracerebral transport occurs at different rates in the white and gray matter (Rosenberg et al., 1980). The glycocalyx of the gray matter has dense synaptic structures that impede the movement of water and other molecules even when the pressure in the ISF is increased (Rosenberg et al., 1982). Molecular movement in gray matter is by diffusion through the extracellular space and bulk flow presumably along vessels. The rate of diffusion of extracellular materials, such as sucose in the gray matter (3.0×10^{-6} cm^2/second) is half that of the same substance in a simple agar gel. The white matter, on the contrary, allows freer movement of water and entrained substances. There are several possible explanations for these differences, including the fact that hyaluronic acid content, which impedes fluid movement, is less in white matter and that white matter fiber tracts are more linear

and cells have fewer synapses so that the diffusion pathways are less tor-
tuous. In addition, blood vessels and their perivascular spaces are less tor-
tuous in white matter. This could allow bulk flow of ISF to occur more
readily in white matter when hydrostatic pressure is increased. This may be
the reason that edema resulting from blood–brain barrier damage, where
extracellular space is enlarged, spreads throughout the white matter of the
brain.

In other species, extracellular transport is more important because of the
lack of a capillary blood–brain barrier. In the elasmobranch family, which
includes the shark and skate, there is a glial rather than an endothelial barrier. Insects also have a glial barrier, whereas lower molluscs have no barrier
(Figure 3–5). Insects have a structured extracellular matrix with acidic glycosaminoglycans and hyaluronic acid. The matrix is important in ion binding
in crustaceans and cephalopods.

Measurements of flow of interstitial fluid have been performed in insects,
Sepia, rat, and cats. Equilibration of tracers between ISF and plasma in the
Sepia brain (C_{isf}/C_{pl}) is less than 1, indicating that the ISF is flowing and
removing the tracer molecules. Calculation of the rate of ISF flow in *Sepia*
is close to the value obtained in the rat (Table 3–5). Abbott et al. (1986)
have suggested that the flow of ISF may be a constant feature of brains with

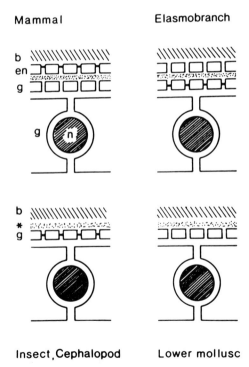

Figure 3–5. The blood–brain barrier in different animals. Layers of the blood–
brain interface: b, blood; en, endothelium; g, glial; n, neuron; stippling, basal lamina. Barrier layer is indicated by bars joining cells. (From Abbott et al., 1986)

Table 3–5. Rate of Flow of Brain Interstitial Fluid in Different Species

Species	Brain ISF Flow (μl/minute)
Sepia (cuttlefish)	0.17–0.19
Rat	0.18–0.29
Rabbit	0.11

From Szentistvanyi et al., 1984, and Abbott et al., 1986.

tight blood–brain interfaces and that control of ISF composition is easier to achieve in a flowing rather than a static milieu.

In higher mammals, the flow of ISF is an important source of CSF. Milhorat (1971) reported that in monkeys with choroid plexuses removed, up to 60 percent of the CSF is produced from ISF. Pollay and Curl (1967) demonstrated CSF formation from the cerebral aqueduct of rabbit. In cat, bulk flow of ISF has been estimated to produce 30 percent of the CSF (Rosenberg et al., 1980). These studies indicate that 30–60 percent of CSF is formed by the ISF and emphasize the importance of extrachoroidal production of CSF in volume regulation in the brain.

Brain sodium, glucose, and amino acids are the primary substances involved in brain volume regulation. Rapid increases in the osmolality of the serum by infusion of hypertonic saline results in the uptake of sodium ions into brain mainly from the CSF (Cserr et al., 1987b). The increase in sodium, however, is less than expected to compensate for the rise in osmolality. Another molecule or series of molecules is formed during hyperosmolar states to balance the increase in serum osmolality. These have been termed "idiogenic osmoles" because the exact identification of the substance involved has proven difficult (Chan and Fishman, 1979; Cserr et al., 1987a). During slow changes in serum osmolality, the idiogenic osmoles develop and prevent damage. However, a rapid rise in serum osmolality without sufficient time to form balancing osmoles leads to the drastic shrinkage of brain tissue and, occasionally, to fatal cerebral hemorrhages.

In a study of the effect of therapeutic doses of mannitol on brain ISF, it was found that the white matter was selectively dehydrated, with a subsequent slowing of ISF transport in white matter (Rosenberg et al., 1988a). Therefore, the gray matter appears to preserve its extracellular volume more easily than does white matter during osmotic changes. This seems reasonable in view of the sensitivity of neurons to ionic changes.

3.5 LYMPHATIC DRAINAGE

ISF performs the function of the lymph of the brain (Bradbury and Cole, 1980). Molecules injected into the caudate nucleus in several animal species drain into the ipsilateral cervical lymphatics (Bradbury et al., 1981). In rabbits, dogs, and sheep, it is suggested that the substances move through the subarachnoid space and across the cribiform plate into the nasal mucosa. However, the significance of this route of ISF drainage in humans is unknown. Dogs normally drain CSF out of the brain into the nasal region (DiChiro et al., 1972). Cats and sheep also have significant drainage by this route. This is a potential route for antigenic fragments of brain tissue to reach the peripheral lymphatics where antibody formation could take place, and the lymphatic drainage in brain may be of importance in autoimmune diseases involving the brain.

Direct injection of ^{131}I-labeled human albumin into the caudate nucleus resulted in greater drainage of the tracer into the ipsilateral lymphatics of the neck (Figure 3–6). When the radiolabeled albumin was injected into CSF, allowing it to move evenly throughout the subarachnoid space, the tracer appeared in both the ipsilateral and countralateral lymph (Bradbury et al., 1981). This suggests that the drainage follows a route within brain tissue that is lateralized and unlikely to involve passage into the CSF in large amounts before it leaves the head.

Clearly, the CNS needs a mechanism to remove substances that may be toxic. Potentially toxic substances released during normal metabolism in-

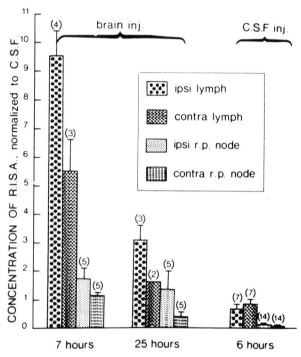

Figure 3–6. Mean concentration of radioiodinated albumin (RISA) in ipsilateral and contralateral deep cervical lymph and in retropharyngeal lymph nodes after intracerebral injection and after single injection into a lateral ventricle of rabbit. Lymph concentration from each experiment was mean of the last 4 half-hour samples. Both lymph and nodal concentration (dpm/mg) have been divided by concentration (dpm/mg) in all CSF obtainable at the end of the experiments. Limits are SE. (From Bradbury et al., 1981)

clude the neurotransmitters, such as glutamate, electrolytes, phospholipases, and plasmin. Also bacteria and viruses can enter the brain. Normally, the substances that are released as part of metabolic processes are taken back into the cell or across the capillary. However, many of them cross the capillary slowly. If they are released in excessive amounts, their removal by ISF would become important. Bacterial and cellular debris are removed by macrophages, and, normally, an occasional macrophage or lymphocyte is seen in the perivascular spaces of the brain (Prineas, 1979).

The basal laminae of cerebral capillaries are composed of collagenous material. They may contribute to the integrity of the blood–brain barrier in several ways. They may form a structural support for the endothelial cell that aids in holding the tight junction in place, they may provide a barrier by their molecular configuration, or they may have a charge and form a charged barrier. Evidence for a role in barrier function comes from the finding that injection of collagenase into the CSF disrupted the blood–brain barrier in rat (Robert and Godeau, 1974). In other organs, such as kidney, pancreas, and intestine, the basement membrane acts as a barrier to certain molecules based on their size and charge. The negatively charged basement membrane may play a similar role in brain, although this remains to be proven experimentally.

3.6 NEUROPEPTIDES AND FLUID HOMEOSTASIS

Neuropeptides, such as arginine vasopressin (AVP) and ANF, influence water movement in the brain. Nerve fibers containing vasopressin project into the brain areas beyond the paraventricular, supraoptic, and suprachiasmatic nuclei of the hypothalamus (Sofroniew and Weindl, 1978). These extrahypothalamic fibers project onto brainstem nuclei, the choroid plexus, cortical regions, and blood vessels. The innervation of blood vessels by vasopressin-containing fibers has been demonstrated by immunohistological studies and by receptor binding assays in isolated microvessels (Kretschmar et al., 1986).

Intravenous injection of high doses of vasopressin increased sodium movement from blood to CSF (Fishman, 1959). Normally, vasopressin appears in picogram/milliliter amounts in the CSF. Since the hormone crosses the blood–brain barrier very slowly, the AVP in the CSF is produced within the CNS. When injected into the CSF of rabbits, AVP lowered CSF pressure by increasing transport of water across the arachnoid villi (Noto et al., 1978). Increased intracranial pressure in humans increased the levels of the hormone in the CSF, suggesting that it may be important in brain edema (Sorensen et al., 1986). Further evidence for a role in brain edema comes from studying cold injury edema, which worsens after vasopressin injection into the CSF (Reeder et al., 1986). These studies performed in animals (using large amounts of the hormone) leave unanswered the question of the role of endogenous vasopressin released in physiological amounts into the brain.

There are numerous stimuli that lead to the release of AVP into the peripheral circulation. Hemorrhage, water deprivation, hypertonic sodium, and hypoxia cause an increase in plasma levels of vasopressin, and hemorrhage, hypoxia, and water deprivation lead to increased levels of the hormone in the CSF. There is a threshold effect with graded hypoxia, with release of hormones occurring only when the oxygen level is lowered to 10 percent of inspired air (Wang et al., 1984). The stimuli that produce release into the periphery are not necessarily the same as those involved in release into the CSF. The CSF has been proposed as the conduit for transport of AVP from the site of release at the median eminence to other regions. However, the release into brain tissue with drainage into CSF also is possible. With current information, it is difficult to decide which of the two mechanisms is active.

Atrial natriuretic peptides are released from cardiac atrial cells. They act on kidney and other peripheral organs to counteract the effect of AVP. Choroid plexus cells have receptors for atriopeptin, and infusion of atriopeptin into the CSF reduced the rate of CSF production by 35 percent (Steardo and Nathanson, 1987). Atriopeptin acts by stimulating the production of cyclic GMP (cGMP), a second messenger. In isolated microvessels, atriopeptin activated guanylate cyclase activity.

Neuropeptides are altered in CSF in several diseases, but the significance of these changes is still unclear. Increased intracranial pressure, such as in pseudotumor cerebri and subarachnoid hemorrhage, increases CSF vasopressin levels (Sorensen, 1986). Hypoxia in animals increases vasopressin levels in both blood and CSF (Wang et al., 1984). A reduced level of CSF somatostatin has been found in Alzheimer's disease (Beal and Martin, 1986).

The mechanism by which vasopressin acts in brain is determined by the receptors to the hormone in brain. Two receptor types have been identified, a V_1 and a V_2 receptor. In rat brain, a V_1 type receptor has been localized to the lateral septum and dorsal hippocampus (Van Leeuwen et al., 1987). Isolated brain capillaries have a V_1 type receptor, and the pial arteries have vasopressin immunoreactive fibers (Itakura et al., 1988).

The V_1 receptor is coupled to a phosphoinositol second messenger system, which in other organs is found near the α-adrenergic receptor. Activation of phosphoinositol results in inositol phosphate (IP_3) and diacylglycerol (DAG) formation. These, in turn, activate protein kinase C (PKC) and the phospholipases. Calcium plays a key role in this process, since it is activated by DAG and augments the phospholipase activation. Phospholipases C and A_2 can release membrane fatty acids, particularly arachidonic acid. Once arachidonic acid and other free fatty acids are formed, they have a series of deleterious effects on cellular function. They inhibit the Na^+, K^+-ATPase and lead to formation of free radicals and leukotrienes, both of which are potent mediators of the inflammatory response. The excessive stimulation of the V_1 receptor on brain cells or blood vessels may play a role in formation of edema, which has been shown to occur with intraventricular injection of AVP (Doczi et al., 1982; Reeder et al., 1986). Edema induced by intracerebral infusion of AVP in cat can be blocked by a V_1 receptor antagonist (Rosenberg et al., 1988b).

REFERENCES

Abbott, N. J., Lane, N. J., Bundgaard, M.: The blood–brain interface in invertebrates. Ann. NY Acad. Sci. 481:20–42, 1986.

Alksne, J. F., Lovings, E. T.: The role of the arachnoid villus in the removal of red blood cells from the subarachnoid space. An electron microscope study in the dog. J. Neurosurg. 36:192–200, 1972.

Ames, A. III, Sakanoue, M., Endo, S.: Na, K, Ca, Mg and Cl concentrations in choroid plexus fluid and cisternal fluid compared with plasma ultrafiltrate. J. Neurophysiol. 27:672–681, 1964.

Beal, M. F., Martin, J. B.: Neuropeptides in neurological disease. Ann. Neurol. 20:547–565, 1986.

Betz, A. L., Goldstein, G. W.: Polarity of the blood–brain barrier: Neutral amino acid transport into isolated brain capillaries. Science 202:225–227, 1978.

Bradbury, M. W., Cole, D. F.: The role of the lymphatic system in drainage of cerebrospinal fluid and aqueous humour. J. Physiol. (Lond) 229:353–365, 1980.

Bradbury, M. W., Cserr, H. F., Westrop, R. J.: Drainage of cerebral interstitial fluid into deep cervical lymph of the rabbit. Am. J. Physiol. 240:329–336, 1981.

Bradbury, M. W. B., Stubbs, J., Hughes, I. E., Parker, P.: The distribution of potassium, sodium, chloride and urea between lumbar cerebrospinal fluid and blood serum in human subjects. Clin. Sci. 25:97–105, 1963.

Brightman, M. W., Reese, T. S.: Junctions between intimately apposed cell membranes in the vertebrate brain. J. Cell. Biol. 40:648–677, 1969.

Chan, P. H., Fishman, R. A.: Elevation of rat brain amino acids, ammonia and idiogenic osmoles induced by hyperosmolality. Brain Res. 161:293–301, 1979.

Crone, C.: The blood–brain barrier as a tight epithelium: Where is information lacking? Ann. NY Acad. Sci. 481:174–185, 1986.

Crone, C., Christensen, O.: Electrical resistance of a capillary endothelium. J. Gen. Physiol. 77:349–371, 1981.

Cserr, H. F.: Physiology of the choroid plexus. Physiol. Rev. 51:273–311, 1971.

Cserr, H. F., Cooper, D. N., Suri, P. K., Patlak, C. S.: Efflux of radiolabeled polyethylene glycols and albumin from rat brain. Am. J. Physiol. 240:319–328, 1981.

Cserr, H. F., DePasquale, M., Patlak, C. S.: Regulation of brain water and electrolytes during acute hyperosmolality in rats. Am. J. Physiol. 253:F522–F529, 1987a.

Cserr, H. F., DePasquale, M., Patlak, C. S.: Volume regulatory influx of electrolytes from plasma to brain during acute hyperosmolality. Am. J. Physiol. 253:F530–F537, 1987b.

Cserr, H. F., Ostrach, L. H.: Bulk flow of interstitial fluid after intracranial injection of blue dextran 2000. Exp. Neurol. 45:50–60, 1974.

Cutler, R. W., Page L., Galicich, J., Watters, G. V.: Formation and absorption of cerebrospinal fluid in man. Brain 91:707–720, 1968.

Davson, H.: *Physiology of the Cerebrospinal Fluid*. London: J & A Churchill, 1967.

Davson, H., Luck, C. P.: The effect of acetazolamide on the chemical composition of the aqueous humour and cerebrospinal fluid and the brain. J. Physiol. (Lond) 137:279–293, 1957.

Davson, H., Pollay, M.: Influence of various drugs on the transport of ^{131}I and PAH across the cerebrospinal fluid–blood barrier. J. Physiol. (Lond) 167:239–246, 1963.

DiChiro, G., Hammock, M. K., Bleyer, W. A.: Spinal descent of cerebrospinal fluid in man. Neurology 26:1–8, 1976.

DiChiro, G., Reames, P. M., Matthews, W. B.: RISA-ventriculography and RISA-cisternography. Neurology 14:185–191, 1964.

DiChiro, G., Stein, S. C., Harrington, T.: Spontaneous cerebrospinal fluid rhinorrhea in normal dogs: Radioisotope studies of an alternate pathway of CSF drainage. J. Neuropathol. Exp. Neurol. 31:447–453, 1972.

Doczi, T., Szerdahelyi, P., Gulya, K., Kiss, J.: Brain water accumulation after the central administration of vasopressin. Neurosurgery 11:402–407, 1982.

Epstein, M. H., Feldman, A. M., Brusilow, S. W.: Cerebrospinal fluid production: Stimulation by cholera toxin. Science 196:1012–1013, 1977.

Fishman, R. A.: Factors influencing the exchange of sodium between plasma and cerebrospinal fluid. J. Clin. Invest. 38:1698–1708, 1959.

Fishman, R. A.: *Cerebrospinal Fluid in Diseases of the Nervous System*. Philadelphia: WB Saunders Company, 1980.

Heisey, S. R., Held, D., Pappenheimer, J. R.: Bulk flow and diffusion in the cerebrospinal fluid system of the goat. Am. J. Physiol. 203:775–781, 1962.

Hussey, F., Schanzer, B. Katzman, R.: A simple constant-infusion manometric test for measurement of CSF absorption. II. Clinical studies, Neurology 20:665–680, 1970.

Itakura, T., Okuno, T., Veno, M., Nakakita, K., Nakai, K., Naka, Y., Imai, H., Kamei, I., Komai, N.: Immunohistochemical demonstration of vasopressin nerve fibers in the cerebral artery. J. Cereb. Blood Flow Metab. 8:606–608, 1988.

Johanson, C. E., Parandoosh, Z., Smith, Q. R.: Cl-HCO$_3$ exchange in choroid plexus: Analysis by the DMO method for cell pH. Am. J. Physiol. 249:F478–F484, 1985.

Katzman, R., Hussey, F.: A simple constant-infusion manometric test for measurement of CSF absorption. I. Rationale and method. Neurology 20:534–544, 1970.

Katzman, R., Pappius, H. M.: *Brain Electrolytes and Fluid Metabolism*. Baltimore: William & Wilkins, 1973.

Kretschmar, R., Landgraf, R., Gjedde, A., Ermisch, A.: Vasopressin binds to microvessels from rat hippocampus. Brain Res. 380:325–330, 1986.

Lane, N. J., Swales, L. S., Abbott, N. J.: Lanthanum penetration in crayfish nervous system: Observations on intact and "desheathed" preparations. J. Cell. Sci. 23:315–324, 1977.

Lindvall, M., Owman, C.: Autonomic nerves in the mammalian choroid plexus and their influence on the formation of cerebrospinal fluid. J. Cereb. Blood Flow Metab. 1:245–266, 1981.

Margolis, R. U., Aquino, D. A., Klinger, M. M., Ripellino, J. A., Margolis, R. K.: Structure and localization of nervous tissue proteoglycans. Ann. NY Acad. Sci. 481:46–54, 1986.

Margolis, R. U., Margolis, R. K.: Metabolism and function of glycoproteins and glycosaminoglycans in nervous tissue. Int. J. Biochem. 8:85–91, 1977.

Masuzawa, T., Sato, F.: The enzyme histochemistry of the choroid plexus. Brain 106:55–99, 1983.

McComb, J. G.: Recent research into the nature of cerebrospinal fluid formation and absorption. J. Neurosurg. 59:369–383, 1983.

Milhorat, T. H.: *Hydrocephalus and the Cerebrospinal Fluid*. Baltimore: Williams & Wilkins, 1972.

Milhorat, T. H., Hammock, M. K., Fenstermacher, J. D., Levin, V. A.: Cerebrospinal fluid production by the choroid plexus and brain. Science 173:330–332, 1971.

Morgulis, S., Perley, A. M.: Studies on cerebrospinal fluid and serum calcium with special reference to the parathyroid hormone. J. Biol. Chem. 88:169–188, 1930.

Murphy, V. A., Smith, Q. R., Rapoport, S. I.: Homeostasis of brain and cerebrospinal fluid calcium concentrations during chronic hypo- and hyperglycemia. J. Neurochem. 47:1735–1741, 1986.

Nathanson, J. A.: Alpha-adrenergic-sensitive adenylate cyclase in choroid plexus: Properties and cellular localization. Mol. Pharmacol. 18:199–209, 1980.

Nicholson, C., Bruggencate, G. T., Steinberg, R., Stockle, H.: Calcium modulation in brain extracellular microenvironment demonstrated with ion-selective micropipette. Proc. Natl. Acad. Sci. USA 74:1287–1290, 1977.

Nicholson, C., Rice, M. E.: Calcium diffusion in the brain cell microenvironment. Can. J. Physiol. Pharmacol. 65:1086–1091, 1987.

Noto, T., Nakajima, T., Saji, Y., Nagawa, Y.: Effect of vasopressin on intracranial pressure of rabbit. Endocrinol. Jpn. 25:591–596, 1978.

Nowak, L., Bregestovski, P., Ascher, P., Herbert, A., Prochianty, A.: Magnesium gates glutamate-activated channels in mouse central neurons. Nature 307:462–465, 1984.

Oldendorf, W. H., Cornford, M. E., Brown, W. J.: The large apparent work capability of the blood–brain barrier: A study of the mitochrondial content of capillary endothelial cells in brain and other tissues of the rat. Ann. Neurol. 1:409–417, 1977.

Olesen, S. P., Crone, C.: Substances that rapidly augment ionic conductance of endothelium in cerebral venules. Acta. Physiol. Scand. 127:233–241, 1986.

Pollay, M.: Formation of cerebrospinal fluid. J. Neurosurg. 42:665–673, 1975.

Pollay, M., Curl, F.: Secretion of cerebrospinal fluid by the ventricular ependyma of the rabbit. Am. J. Physiol. 213:1031–1038, 1967.

Prineas, J. W.: Multiple sclerosis: Presence of lymphatic capillaries and lymphoid tissue in the brain and spinal cord. Science 203:1123–1125, 1979.

Pullen, R. G. L., DePasquale, M., Cserr, H. F.: Bulk flow of cerebrospinal fluid into brain in response to acute hyperosmolality. Am. J. Physiol. 253:F538–F545, 1987.

Rapoport, S. I.: *Blood–Brain Barrier in Physiology and Medicine*. New York: Raven Press, 1976.

Reeder, R. F., Nattie, E. E., North, W. G.: Effect of vasopressin on cold-induced brain edema in cats. J. Neurosurg. 64:941–950, 1986.

Rennels, M. L., Gregory, T. F., Blaumanis, O. R., Fujimoto, K., Grady, P. A.: Evidence for a "paravascular" fluid circulation in the mammalian central nervous system, provided by the rapid distribution of tracer protein throughout the brain from the subarachnoid space. Brain Res. 326:47–63, 1985.

Robert, A. M., Godeau, G.: Action of proteolytic and glycolytic enzymes on the permeability of the blood–brain barrier. Biomedicine 21:36–39, 1974.

Rosenberg, G. A., Barrett, J., Estrada, E., Brayer, J., Kyner, W. T.: Selective effect of mannitol-induced hyperosmolality on brain interstitial fluid and water content in white matter. Metab. Brain Dis. 3:217–227, 1988a.

Rosenberg, G. A., Estrada, E., Kyner, W. T.: The effect of arginine vasopressin and V₁ receptor antagonist on brain water in cat. Neurosci. Lett. 95:241–245, 1988b.

Rosenberg, G. A., Kyner, W. T., Estrada, E.: Bulk flow of brain interstitial fluid under normal and hyperosmolar conditions. Am. J. Physiol. 238:42–49, 1980.

Rosenberg, G. A., Kyner, W. T., Estrada, E.: The effect of increased CSF pressure on interstitial fluid flow during ventriculocisternal perfusion in the cat. Brain Res. 232:141–150, 1982.

Rosenberg, G. A., Kyner, W. T., Fenstermacher, J. D., Patlak, C. S.: Effect of vasopressin on ependymal and capillary permeability to tritiated water in cat. Am. J. Physiol. 251:F485–F489, 1986.

Rosenberg, G. A., Wolfson, L., Katzman, R.: Pressure-dependent bulk flow of cerebrospinal fluid into brain. Exp. Neurol. 60:267–276, 1978.

Rothman, S. M., Olney, J. W.: Glutamate and the pathophysiology of hypoxic–ischemic brain damage. Ann. Neurol. 19:105–111, 1986.

Sahar, A., Tsipstein, E.: Effects of mannitol and furosemide on the rate of formation of cerebrospinal fluid. Exp. Neurol. 60:584–591, 1978.

Saito, Y., Wright, E. M.: Bicarbonate transport across the frog choroid plexus and its control by cyclic nucleotides. J. Physiol. (Lond) 336:635–648, 1983.

Siesjo, B. K.: Historical overview: Calcium, ischemia, and death of brain cells. Ann. NY Acad. Sci. 522:638–661, 1988.

Smith, Q. R., Rapoport, S. I.: Cerebrovascular permeability coefficients to sodium, potassium, and chloride. J. Neurochem. 46:1732–1742, 1986.

Sofroniew, M. V., Weindl, A.: Projections from the parvocellular vasopressin- and neurophysin-containing neurons of the suprachiasmatic nucleus. Am. J. Anat. 153:391–429, 1978.

Sorenson, P. S.: Studies of vasopressin in human cerebrospinal fluid. Acta. Neurol. Scand. 74:81–102, 1986.

Steardo, L., Nathanson, J. A.: Brain barrier tissues: End-organs for atriopeptins. Science 235:470–473, 1987.

Szentistvanyi, I., Patlak, C. S., Ellis, R. A., Cserr, H. F.: Drainage of interstitial fluid from different regions of rat brain. Am. J. Physiol. 246:F835–F844, 1984.

Tai, C. Y., Smith, Q. R., Rapoport, S. I.: Calcium influxes into brain and cerebrospinal fluid are linearly related to plasma ionized calcium concentration. Brain Res. 385:227–236, 1986.

Tripathi, B. J., Tripathi, R. C.: Vacuolar transcellular channels as a drainage pathway for cerebrospinal fluid. J. Physiol. (Lond) 239:195–206, 1974.

van Leeuwen, F. W., van der Beek, E. M., van Heerikhuize, J. J., Wolters, P., van der Meulen, G., Wan, W. P.: Quantitative light microscopic autoradiographic localization of binding sites labelled with [³H] vasopressin antagonist d(CH₂)₅[Tyr(Me)²]VP in the rat brain, pituitary and kidney. Neurosci. Lett. 80:121–126, 1987.

Wang, B. C., Sundet, W. D., Goetz, K. L.: Vasopressin in plasma and cerebrospinal fluid of dogs during hypoxia or acidosis. Am. J. Physiol. 247:E449–55, 1984.

Wang, H. H., Adey, W. R.: Effects of cations and hyaluronidase on cerebral electrical impedence. Exp. Neurol. 25:70–84, 1969.

Weed, L. H.: Studies on cerebrospinal fluid IV. The dual source of cerebrospinal fluid. J. Med. Res. 31:93–117, 1914.

Weed, L. H.: Certain anatomical and physiological aspects of the meninges and cerebrospinal fluid. Brain 58:383–397, 1935.

Welch, K., Friedman, V.: The cerebrospinal fluid values. Brain 83:454–469, 1960.

Wise, B. L., Chater, N.: The value of hypertonic mannitol solution in decreasing brain mass and lowering cerebrospinal fluid pressure. J. Neurosurg. 19:1038–1043, 1962.

Wong, R. P. K., Bradbury, M. W. B.: Permeability of the blood–brain barrier to calcium in adrenal insufficiency. Brain Res. 84:361–364, 1975.

Woodbury, J., Lyons, K., Carretta, R., Hahn, A., Sullivan, J. F.: Cerebrospinal fluid and serum levels of magnesium, zinc, and calcium in man. Neurology 18:700–705, 1968.

4

Mathematics of Transport

4.1 INTRODUCTION

Several methods have been used to analyze the transport of various substances from blood to brain. Qualitative information about the integrity of the blood-brain barrier after pathological alterations can be obtained relatively simply by the use of dyes that stain brain tissue after their entrance from the blood to the brain. The most commonly used dye is Evans blue, which binds to albumin and stains the brain in regions with altered barrier function. Quantitative measurements of blood to brain transport across the capillary can be done by the injection of a very small or tracer amount of a radiolabeled molecule. A number of tracer methods have been devised, and each has its advantages and drawbacks.

The qualitative and quantitative methods fall into several major categories. In some cases, there is both qualitative and quantitative information depending on the method of measurement. For example, Evans blue is a visual marker of barrier damage, but it can provide quantitative information if the content of dye is measured quantitatively in brain tissue. Another example is the qualitative information about receptor binding in humans that is available with the gamma-emitting substances measured with single photon emission tomography. When the same substance is labeled with a positron-emitting substance and measured with PET, it is possible to obtain quantitative information. The main methods used to study blood-brain barrier transport are listed in Table 4–1.

Clinically, the integrity of the blood-brain barrier can be studied with CT by the intravenous infusion of a radiopaque contrast agent containing iodide. If the barrier is disrupted, the contrast agent will be seen within the brain tissue. MRI can be enhanced by the intravenous infusion of gadolinium (Gd)-DTPA. The paramagnetic properties of gadolinium shorten the relaxation

Table 4-1. Methods for Measurement of Blood-Brain Barrier Permeability

Qualitative Methods	Quantitative Methods
Dye injection (Evans blue)	Indicator dilution
Constrast enhancement in CT and MRI	Brain uptake
Isotopic brain scans	Single-injection external registration
	Intravenous infusion

time for water, which enhances the T_1-weighted image. Normally, both the contrast agents seen by CT and the paramagnetic agents used in MRI are present only in the vascular spaces of the brain. CT and MRI have replaced to a large extent brain scanning with gamma-ray emitting agents. Another recently developed imaging method, PET, allows both the visualization of a positron-emitting species of rubidium and the measurement of the rate of its transport from the blood to the brain. Rubidium acts the same as potassium and normally is excluded from the brain.

The quantitative methods that have been used primarily in animals fall into several categories: indicator dilution (Crone, 1965), brain uptake (Oldendorf, 1970), single-injection external registration (Raichle et al., 1976), intravenous administration (Davson and Segal, 1970; Davson and Welch, 1971; Daniel et al., 1977; Ohno et al., 1978), and in situ brain perfusion (Takasato et al., 1984). Most of the information currently available on capillary transport has been obtained with these methods.

The choice of the method depends on the type of information desired and the characteristics of the substance studied. Methods that use a carotid injection and measure a single passage through the brain are excellent for rapidly transported substances but are too insensitive to detect those that are more slowly transported. For the more slowly transported molecules, intravenous infusion of a bolus or an amount to maintain a steady blood level can be used. Some methods use blood entering and leaving the brain so that they provide whole brain measurements, whereas others can be done with autoradiograms or tomography and yield regional information. Finally, some substances are so rapidly transported out of the blood into the brain that they can serve as markers of blood flow. Thus, the problem to be analyzed determines the most appropriate method for its analysis.

Crone (1965) showed that glucose enters brain by carrier-mediated transport. He called his method "indicator dilution" because the tracer molecule is diluted by the blood while an impermeable indicator molecule, added to correct for the amount of dilution, remains in the blood. In brief, the movement into brain of a diffusible test substance is determined by sampling blood at the sagittal sinus and comparing the concentration of the test substance in the efflux with its concentration in the infused solution and then comparing both efflux and influx of the test substance to that of the nondiffusible marker substance. Oldendorf (1970) modified the indicator dilution method and measured brain uptake of a rapidly diffusible ^{3}H-labeled reference substance and a less diffusible test substance labeled with [14]C. Another approach was developed by Davson (1967) that used the steady-state intravenous infusion of a radiolabeled test substance with an infusion apparatus that maintained a constant blood level (Davson and Segal, 1970; Davson et al., 1971; Daniel et al., 1977). Davson used his method to study less permeable substances, such as sodium, that require a longer time to enter the brain. A modification of the intravenous method that uses a bolus intravenous injection also has been used to measure transport of substances with low permeability and little backflux (Ohno et al., 1978). A further modification involving in situ external carotid perfusion is useful for molecules of intermediate permeability, such as amino acids (Takasato et al., 1984).

4.2 SINGLE-INJECTION METHODS

Permeability of a membrane to a given substance is the rate at which that substance crosses the membrane. Although permeability is a complex function of the membrane structure and the reaction of the membrane to the substance, a functional definition relates the rate of movement across the membrane to the concentration of the substance on either side. Both impermeable and permeable substances are diluted by the blood when they are injected into the carotid. However, permeable molecules diffuse across the endothelial cell membrane to enter the brain and CSF. Therefore, after injection into the carotid artery, if both the arterial concentration and the venous concentration as sampled at the sagittal sinus are known, the amount extracted during passage through the brain can be calculated. In other words, injecting into the carotid and sampling at the sagittal sinus gives the arteriovenous (AV) difference.

The amount of a substance extracted by the brain (E) as the blood flows through the region is defined as the AV difference divided by the arterial concentration.

$$E = \frac{(C_a - C_v)}{C_a} \tag{4-1}$$

or

$$E = 1 - \left(\frac{C_v}{C_a}\right) \tag{4-2}$$

where C_v equals venous concentration and C_a equals arterial concentration. After injection, dilution occurs, and the arterial concentration is unknown. Since both test and reference substances are equally diluted, the ratio of the concentration of the permeable test substance to that of the impermeable reference substance in the injection fluid is known and remains constant. However, removal of the permeable test substance by the brain changes the ratio of test and reference substances in the venous blood. Thus, ratios rather than absolute amounts reflect the amount of test substance lost to the brain. Knowing the concentrations of the test and indicator substances in both the injectate and the venous outflow provides sufficient information to calculate the amount extracted (Figure 4–1).

Flux relates the extraction value to permeability of the membrane. It is the product of flow through a surface and the concentration. It has the units of amount per time. Permeability (P) is defined by the flux, the surface area (A), and the change in concentration, dC, using the relationship

$$P = \frac{flux}{A \times dC} \tag{4-3}$$

The units for permeability are cm/second. Another way of expressing the flux is by blood flow. The flux equals the blood flow (F) through the vessel and the arteriovenous difference, i.e., the arterial concentration, C_a, and the venous concentration, C_v:

$$Flux = F(C_a - C_v) \tag{4-4}$$

leading to the relationship

$$PA = \frac{F(C_a - C_v)}{dC} \tag{4-5}$$

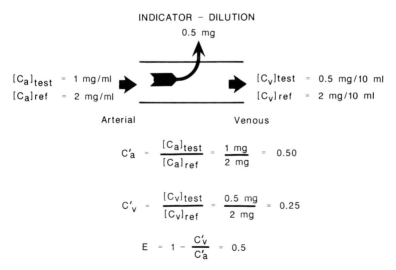

Figure 4–1. Illustrative example of the calculation of the extraction fraction (E) using the indicator dilution method with a partially permeable, extracted test substance of concentration $[C_a]_{test}$ in the artery and an impermeable reference substance $[C_a]_{ref}$.

The change in concentration is not known, and Crone (1965) estimated it empirically with the relationship

$$dC = \frac{(C_a - C_v)}{[\ln (C_a/C_v)]} \qquad (4\text{--}6)$$

Substituting this into the earlier equation gives

$$PA = -F \ln (1 - E) \qquad (4\text{--}7)$$

The flow and the extraction rate can be estimated or experimentally determined so that the permeability of the surface area can be calculated. Estimating the surface area allows calculation of the permeability itself. The indicator dilution method is best suited for repeated measurements of moderately permeable molecules, such as glucose. Limitations of the method include extracerebral contamination of sinus blood, changes in blood flow by the injection, and lack of regional specificity. Studies in humans have been done with the indicator dilution method. Sampling of venous blood is done at the jugular bulb, and, therefore, these studies require catheter placement in the carotid artery and jugular vein, which limits the use of this method clinically to a few research centers.

4.3 BRAIN UPTAKE INDEX

Oldendorf (1970) developed an intraarterial injection method for use in animals that compared brain uptake of a rapidly diffusible reference molecule with that of a less permeable test substance (Figure 4–2). Fifteen seconds after injection of the tracers into the carotid, the brain is removed, and the amounts of both the test and the reference substances in brain are measured. Ratios of the test substance to the reference substance in both the brain and the blood can be measured. A brain uptake index (BUI) can be calculated by the expression

$$BUI = (C_t/C_r)_{br}/(C_t/C_r)_{inj} \times 100 \qquad (4\text{--}8)$$

where C_t is concentration of the test substance and C_r is concentration of the reference compound either in the brain or in the injectate. Generally, the reference molecule is ^{3}H-labeled water, and the test substance is a ^{14}C-labeled compound.

Ideally, the reference substance would be completely extracted in a single passage through the brain in order to be able to calculate an accurate value for extraction of the test substance. A less permeable reference substance would lower its concentration in the brain and falsely elevate the BUI (Bradbury et al., 1975). Although water diffuses rapidly across the endothelial cell, its uptake is limited by its diffusion across the capillary (diffusion lim-

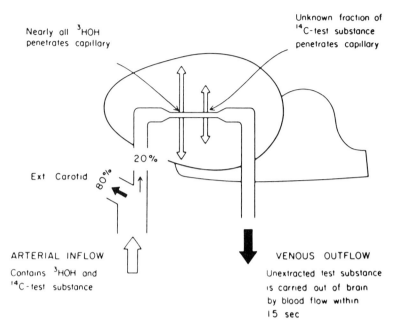

Figure 4–2. Diagram of brain uptake index method. A buffered solution containing a ^{14}C-labeled test solute and $^{3}H_2O$ is injected into the common carotid artery of a rat, an the animal is decapitated 15 second later. (From Oldendorf, 1981)

itation) (Raichle et al., 1974). The slower than expected diffusion rate makes the amount of water extracted dependent on the rate of cerebral blood flow. This can present a problem, since intracarotid injection may alter the blood flow. In fact, the carotid injection of a 200 μl bolus in less than 1 second alters blood flow. To overcome the problem caused by the diffusion limitation of water, ^{14}C-butanol has been used as the reference tracer because it is more rapidly transported. In spite of the flow limitation, very useful information has been obtained using the BUI method. For most molecules, the effect of water limitation is minimal, and for those where it is a problem, corrections can be made for the lower extraction rate. Therefore, the BUI method has been used to study the moderately permeable molecules, such as the narcotics, the peptides, and the amino acids.

Conversion of BUI to E can be done assuming that there is negligible backflux of test tracer, using the formula

$$E = \frac{c \, BUI}{100} \qquad (4\text{--}9)$$

where c is a constant that depends on blood flow, the reference tracer, decapitation time, and brain region sampled. An estimate of PA is then obtainable with Equation 4–7. The BUI method has been used extensively because it is relatively simple to perform. However, translation of BUI to PA has been hampered by the need to determine the constants.

Although it is appealing to express the movement of a test substance from the blood to the brain in terms of permeability, the inability to measure the surface area directly introduces considerable uncertainty into the measurement. Capillary surface area has been estimated for different brain regions. The capillary is a dynamic structure that undergoes changes in its surface area in response to changes in its environment. Therefore, the combined expression for permeability and surface area should be used unless the surface area can be unambiguously determined.

4.4 SINGLE-INJECTION EXTERNAL REGISTRATION

A method to measure capillary permeability is the intracarotid or intravenous injection of a short-lived radioisotope that is rapidly taken up by the brain and can be sensed by an external detector (Raichle et al., 1974; Raichle et al., 1976). A positron-labeled substance, such as ^{15}O-labeled water or ^{11}C-labeled carbon monoxide, is injected into the carotid or intravenously. External detectors register the appearance of the tracer in the head and its clearance. Since water is rapidly transported, it serves as a useful estimate of the rate of blood flow (its slight diffusion limitation results in an underestimation in high-flow states). This method has been used to show changes in water permeability induced by various agents, including vasopressin, locus coeruleus stimulation, and osmotic agents.

4.5 COMPARTMENTAL APPROACH TO INTRAVENOUS INFUSION

Davson (1967) demonstrated the low capillary permeability of sodium ions by controlling the concentration of the ion in the blood. He calculated transfer constants using a first-order differential equation for a two-compartment system. This method is useful to study molecules that are slowly permeable and have little backflux from brain to blood during the time of infusion.

Transport of a substance from blood to brain results in a buildup in the brain compartment and backflux in the opposite direction. A two-compartment model that incorporates blood flow has been developed by Rapoport et al. (1979):

$$dC_{br}/dt = k(C_{pl} - C_{br}/V_{br}) \qquad (4-10)$$

where C_{br} is the brain concentration of the tracer, C_{pl} is the arterial concentration, V_{br} is the volume fraction within which the substance is distributed, and t is time.

Fick's equation and conservation of mass can be employed to define the constant, k, which is related to blood flow (F) and permeability (P) for a given surface area (A) by the equation (Smith, 1985)

$$k = F[1 - e^{(-PA/F)}] \qquad (4\text{--}11)$$

When backflux is negligible, $C_{br}/V_{br} = 0$ and the equations reduce to

$$dC_{br}/dt = k\,C_{pl} \qquad (4\text{--}12)$$

So that at time (T), assuming the brain concentration of the substance equals zero, $[C_{br}(0) = 0]$

$$C_{br} = k \int_0^T C_{pl}dt \qquad (4\text{--}13)$$

which, by substituting from Equations 4–7 and 4–11, becomes

$$PA = -F\ln\left[1 - \left(C_{br}(T)/F \int_0^T C_{pl}dt\right)\right] \qquad (4\text{--}14)$$

The intravenous bolus injection method is best suited for substances that are slowly permeable. The method requires multiple blood samples during the experiment and removal of the brain at the end of the experiment. Sucrose, mannitol, neuropeptides, chemotherapeutic agents, and other relatively impermeable substances have been measured with this technique. A correction is needed for the volume of blood in brain to correct for isotope remaining in the blood. This is done in other animals using short injection times with the formula

$$C_{br}(t) = C_t(t) - VC_{bl}(t) \qquad (4\text{--}15)$$

where $C_{br}(t)$ is concentration in brain, and $C_{bl}(t)$ is concentration in blood, $C_t(t)$ is the total tracer concentration, and V is fractional volume of blood. Blood volumes generally range from 1 to 2 percent in most brain regions. An alternative method is to use a second tracer that does not cross the blood–brain barrier as an indication of vascular volume. This could be a large radiolabeled molecule, such as inulin, dextran, or albumin.

When the backflux is significant, a two-compartment analysis is needed. For some substances, transport into the CSF compartment also may be important and a three-compartment model is needed. The concentration in the blood may vary in a complicated manner. For accurate studies with variable plasma levels, multiple time points are needed, and a computer with a nonlinear regression program becomes necessary for data analysis. Fortunately, for most compounds and study times, the simple one- or two-compartment model is sufficient.

Regional studies of blood–brain barrier transport are of interest in the study of pathological processes, such as brain tumors, injury, and experimental allergic encephalomyelitis. Aminoisobutyric (AIB) acid is an amino acid that is passively transported into brain. Normally, its transport is slow, but in pathological conditions, the rate is increased. An autoradiographic method for blood to brain transfer using AIB has been developed that has been used to study pathological processes (Blasberg et al., 1983). The amino acid concentration in blood is recorded at multiple points after its intravenous injection. After a given time period, the brain is removed, frozen, and prepared for autoradiography. The AIB method is excellent for analysis of pathological states, since under normal conditions it is very slowly taken up by brain.

In some circumstances, it is useful to control the concentration in the plasma very carefully for an extended period of time. When a steady-state is achieved in the blood, the time variant part of the differential equation is greatly simplified. This is difficult in the intact animal because of the loss of substrate to other organs, such as the kidney and liver. Isolation of the brain circulation allows direct perfusion of the brain with the substance under study. Complete isolation of the circulation requires extensive surgical manipulation. To perfuse the hemisphere for up to 5 minutes, use of the external carotid is possible. An in situ perfusion method has been described involving cannulation of the external carotid and perfusion of a hemisphere for 5–300 seconds (Takasato et al., 1984). This allows longer time periods than single-injection methods, which are limited to 5–15 seconds. The perfusate totally replaces blood for the perfusion period. Permeability constants are calculated by compartmental equations, assuming no backflux. The in situ method, like the intravenous infusion method, can be used to measure relatively impermeable molecules and, in addition, allows manipulation of the perfusion fluid. Surgical preparation and regulation of infusion parameters are more complicated in the in situ method than with intravenous injection (Figure 4–3).

4.6 QUALITATIVE PERMEABILITY MEASURES

There are both laboratory and clinical techniques to demonstrate abnormal capillary permeability. In animals, the injection of a large dye molecule that remains in the blood except under pathological conditions commonly is employed. For example, in a study of the effect of carotid artery occlusion in the gerbil, the extent of damage from the stroke was determined behaviorally and correlated to the extent of the damage as observed histologically. The integrity of the blood–brain barrier was determined by the injection of the dye, Evans blue, before the animal was killed. Quantitative data were obtained by homogenizing the brain and measuring its concentration of Evans blue by fluorescence spectrophotometry (Uyama et al., 1988).

Contrast agents for use in CT and MRI provide a clinical method to assess barrier function. Iodide-labeled contrast agents are radiopaque to x-rays. When injected into the blood, they remain within the vasculature except when the blood–brain barrier is abnormal. Brain lesions show up as regions of in-

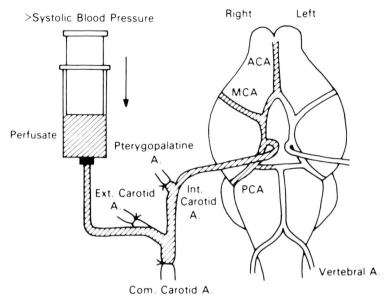

Figure 4–3. Diagram of technique for perfusing the right cerebral hemisphere of a rat. ACA, anterior cerebral artery; MCA, middle cerebral artery; PCA, posterior cerebral artery. (From Takasato et al., 1984)

creased density on the CT scan. An MRI contrast agent, Gd-DTPA, alters the magnetic characteristics of the tissue. Therefore, if the barrier is damaged, the Gd-DTPA enters the brain and enhances the proton signal. Contrast agents are extremely important in CT diagnosis; they show increased permeability of brain tumors, abscesses, acute demyelination, and vascular malformations. The role of contrast agents in MRI is less clearly defined. Gadolinium has been studied experimentally, but its role in clinical diagnosis is under investigation.

4.7 CARRIER-MEDIATED TRANSPORT

Essential nutrients, such as glucose and the amino acids, cross the blood–brain barrier by carrier-mediated transport. The characteristic of carrier-mediated transport is that it can be saturated as the concentration of the substrate increases to reach a maximum. At that point, the transport follows the pattern of diffusive movement. The mathematical formulation of a carrier system is based on the Michaelis–Menten equations for enzymes. In enzyme terminology

$$E_z + S \underset{k_{-1}}{\overset{k_1}{\rightleftharpoons}} C \underset{k_{-2}}{\overset{k_2}{\rightleftharpoons}} E_z + P \qquad (4\text{–}16)$$

The enzyme, E_z, combines with substrate S to form the carrier complex, C, which gives the enzyme back plus the product, P. The Michaelis–Menten enzyme kinetic type equation used to describe the rate of the above reaction V_0 is

$$V_0 = k_2 E_0 S_0 / [S_0 + (k_{-1} + k_1)/k_1] \qquad (4\text{--}17)$$

If the term V_{max} is set equal to $k_2 E_0$ and K_m is equal to $(k_{-1} + k_2)/k_1$, then the final relationship is

$$V_0 = V_{max} S_0 / (S_0 + K_m) \qquad (4\text{--}18)$$

where V_{max} is interpreted to be the maximum rate of transport.

Michaelis–Menten constants have been calculated from the indicator dilution methods (Betz and Iannotti, 1983) and the brain uptake index (Pardridge, 1983). The rate of glucose uptake is determined from the arterial glucose concentration, C_a, the rate of cerebral blood flow, F, and the extraction, E, which is the amount of ^{14}C-labeled material taken up by brain after intracarotid injection, with tritiated water as the reference. The rate of unidirectional influx, V, is

$$V = EFC_a \qquad (4\text{--}19)$$

where V is in units, such as $\mu mol\ min^{-1}\ g^{-1}$. By analogy to the Michaelis–Menten equation for enzyme kinetics, the influx can be calculated. Because some of the transport occurs by diffusion unrelated to the carrier, a diffusion term is added to the equation:

$$V = [V_{max} C_a / (K_m + C_a)] + K_d C_a \qquad (4\text{--}20)$$

where K_d is the nonsaturable transport constant related to diffusion. Several methods are available to derive the constants from the experimental data with Equation 4–20. However, the need to determine K_m, V_{max}, and K_d from a few data points and the different ways of performing the computation have led to differences in the literature for the various values.

The kinetic equation can be related to the extraction and the permeability:

$$E = PA/F \qquad (4\text{--}21)$$

so that

$$PA = [V_{max}/(K_m + C_a)] + K_d \qquad (4\text{--}22)$$

Using Equation 4–7 (note that extraction E is uptake rather than dilution and that when E is small, $\ln(1 - E) \approx -E$), E becomes

$$E = 1 - e^{(-PA/F)} \tag{4-23}$$

leading to the general expression

$$E = 1 - e^{(-[V_{max}/(K_m+C_a)+K_d]/F)} \tag{4-24}$$

which can be solved for the parameters V_{max}, K_m and K_d by nonlinear regression analysis methods.

4.8 CEREBRAL BLOOD FLOW: SCHMIDT-KETY APPROACH

The brain receives a disproportionate amount of the total blood flow to the body. Because of the constant need of the brain for oxygen and glucose, interruption of blood flow impairs consciousness and, if prolonged for over 5 minutes, can lead to irreversible cell damage. Output from the heart is regulated to ensure a steady supply of blood to the brain. Besides cardiac regulation, the cerebral vasculature has autoregulatory mechanisms. A fall in blood pressure dilates vessels, whereas an increase in pressure vasoconstricts them. Complex biochemical events are involved in regulation of blood flow.

Measurement of cerebral blood flow (CBF) was made using Fick's law, which states that the change in the amount of a substance, m, within a given volume, v, is equal to the amount entering the volume, J_{in}, minus the amount leaving, J_{out}, so that

$$dm/dt = J_{in} - J_{out} \tag{4-25}$$

For oxygen, the amount entering a tissue is equal to the blood flow, F, times the arterial concentration, C_a. Likewise, the amount leaving is the flow times the venous concentration, C_v. If Q is the quantity at time, t, then

$$dQ/dt = F(C_a - C_v) \tag{4-26}$$

When blood flow to an organ is known from a separate determination, the oxygen consumption of that organ can be determined. On the other hand, when the substance is not metabolized, it can be used to measure blood flow (Kety and Schmidt, 1948). The anesthetic agent, nitrous oxide, is an inert gas that can be inhaled in amounts lower than used to produce the anesthetic effect and that equilibrates with brain tissue in 10–15 minutes. The arterial concentration can be sampled, and the venous concentration coming from the brain can be obtained from the jugular bulb.

The mass conservation equation for a substance that is metabolized is given by

$$Q_a = Q_v + Q_m + Q_i \tag{4-27}$$

where Q_a is the amount in the artery, Q_v is the amount in the vein, Q_m is the metabolized portion, and Q_i is the amount taken up by the organ. For oxygen, which is practically all metabolized, $Q_i = 0$, whereas for nitrous oxide, which is inert, $Q_m = 0$. The amount taken up is the product of the flow to the organ and the concentration:

$$Q = F \times C \qquad (4\text{--}28)$$

and for nitrous oxide

$$dQ_i/dt = F(C_a - C_v) \qquad (4\text{--}29)$$

so that

$$F = Q_i(T) \Big/ \int_0^T (C_a - C_v)dt \qquad (4\text{--}30)$$

At equilibrium, part of the gas is in the brain and part is in the blood. In a given amount of brain tissue, there is a quantity of gas equal to $Q_i(T)$ at time T. The amount in the brain can be estimated from the venous concentration by the so-called partition coefficient (α). This is necessary because the actual amount of nitrous oxide in brain tissue cannot be measured. Nitrous oxide is a marker of blood flow because it has a partition coefficient of 1. By definition, the

$$\alpha_{N_2O} = [(Q_i(T)/W)]/C_v(T) \qquad (4\text{--}31)$$

Since $\alpha = 1$, when time is infinite, $C_v(T)$ is the amount in the brain, which when multiplied by the weight, W, equals the amount, so that

$$F = C_v(T)W \Big/ \int_0^T (C_a - C_v)dt \qquad (4\text{--}32)$$

The CBF for a given weight is the flow divided by the weight, F/W.

The measurement of CBF can be made in people. The subject inhales 15 percent N_2O, and its concentration in the arterial blood and the jugular bulb is sampled at multiple time points over 10 minutes. The integrals of the arteriovenous difference and the CBF are calculated. Equation 4–32 pertains to any substance that rapidly passes the blood–brain barrier.

The nitrous oxide method, which provides a value for blood flow to the entire brain rather than the regional flow, was used initially to determine normal CBF in healthy volunteers as well as the effects of various diseases.

4.9 REGIONAL BLOOD FLOW

Methods to measure regional cerebral flow were developed based on the Kety-Schmidt approach but using tracers rapidly transported into brain. A xenon radioisotopic method was developed for use with external radiation detectors, and an autoradiographic method was developed for use in experimental animals. The essential feature of the regional method is the ability to measure a substance both in the brain region of interest and in the blood. The equations are similar to those for the nitrous oxide method, except the concentration of the substance in the vein (C_v) is estimated from the partition coefficient, α_i, and the brain concentration (C_i) in a region, i

$$C_v = C_i/\alpha_i \qquad (4\text{--}33)$$

so that the basic Equation 4–29 becomes

$$dC_i/dt = (F_i/W_i)(C_a - C_i/\alpha_i) \qquad (4\text{--}34)$$

and if a constant is defined by

$$k_i = F_i/\alpha_i W_i \qquad (4\text{--}35)$$

then

$$dC_i/dt = k_i(\alpha_i C_a - C_i) \qquad (4\text{--}36)$$

and

$$dC_i/dt = -k_i C_i + \alpha_i k_i C_a \qquad (4\text{--}37)$$

and a solution to this differential equation is

$$C_i(T) = \alpha_i k_i \int_0^T C_a e^{[-k_i(T-t)]}dt \qquad (4\text{--}38)$$

Several substances have been used to measure blood flow by autoradiography. The one that has proven most useful is ^{14}C-iodoantipyrine, which has a partition coefficient of 0.8 (Sakurada et al., 1978). The tracer is injected intravenously and sampled arterially multiple times for several minutes, at which time the brain is rapidly removed for autoradiography. From the final concentration in the blood and the amount in the various brain regions, the rate of blood flow is determined.

4.10 HYDROGEN CLEARANCE METHOD

An alternative method for measurement of blood flow in a single region is based on the fact that hydrogen gas changes the electrical properties of platinum wire. The change in resistance in the wire is recorded on a polygraph, and these changes can be used to calculate CBF.

A platinum electrode is implanted in the region of the brain where blood flow is to be measured. Hydrogen gas in 5–7 percent concentration is inhaled while the electrical currents are measured from the electrode. When a steady-state is reached, the gas is stopped and the washout of the gas corresponds to the return of the electrical signal to baseline. The rate at which the gas is cleared from the region is a measure of the blood flow.

Hydrogen clearance is an excellent method to follow blood flow over time, since multiple measurements can be taken over a relatively short time frame, but it is invasive and limited to several regions (Symon et al., 1974). However, it overcomes the ability to obtain only one point in time as is done with autoradiographic and tissue sampling methods. Other substances also can be used as markers of clearance. Xenon with CT and radioactive xenon with external detectors are two examples. Inhaled radioactive xenon has been used, but with it there is the problem of contamination from the external carotid circulation.

Clearance equations are expressed as exponentials:

$$C_i(T) = C_0 e^{-k_i T} \qquad\qquad (4\text{--}39)$$

where C_0 is the initial tissue concentration, and the decay constant k_i represents the rate of clearance of the gas. Unless the tissue is pure gray or white matter, there are two clearance curves; one is a steep curve for fast flow gray matter component, and the other is a less steep curve for the slower white matter.

Another method that can be used to obtain multiple time points is the use of labeled microspheres. Differently labeled spheres can be injected at various time points. Up to 5 different radioactive labels have been possible to count. This method is very useful if measurements in regions are needed during several different experimental states, such as before, during, and after vascular occlusion.

4.11 INTRACEREBRAL TRANSPORT

The movement of molecules between cells and along perivascular spaces can be measured with radiolabeled extracellular markers. When a molecule in solution is placed in contact with a porous substance, it moves into that substance by diffusion and by bulk flow. The basic equations describing the movement into tissue by molecules in a fluid bathing the tissue's surface are derived from those used to describe the transfer of heat between two substances and from those for convexity flow.

To measure the movement into brain tissue, it is necessary to maintain a constant concentration of the substance bathing the surface. This can be done by the ventriculocisternal perfusion technique (Pappenheimer et al., 1962). An inflow needle is implanted stereotactically into the lateral ventricle, and an outflow needle is inserted into the cisterna magna. An isotopically labeled extracellular molecule is perfused through the ventricles, and the brain is removed for analysis. Sections are made from the surface inward at known distances from the surface. From the radioactive content in the tissue at different depths from the surface, the diffusion coefficients can be calculated.

The formula for calculation of the diffusion coefficients in one dimension is

$$C(x,t) = C_0 \cdot \text{erfc}(x/2\sqrt{D_A t}) \tag{4-40}$$

where erfc is the error function. This equation can be solved for the apparent diffusion coefficient, D_A, and for the extracellular space, C_0. The rate of diffusion across the ependymal surface has been calculated for radiolabeled sucrose and inulin (Rall et al., 1962; Katzman et al., 1968; Patlak and Fenstermacher, 1975).

In addition to diffusion, there is bulk flow in tissue. The rate of bulk flow can be determined along with the diffusion coefficient by a parameter estimation method (Rosenberg et al., 1980). The equation for calculation of both diffusion and bulk flow is

$$C(x,t) = \frac{C_0}{2}\left\{\text{erfc}\left(\frac{x - Vt}{2\sqrt{Dt}}\right) + e^{\left(\frac{xV}{D}\right)}\text{erfc}\left(\frac{x + Vt}{2\sqrt{Dt}}\right)\right\} \tag{4-41}$$

Calculation of diffusion coefficients has been done for agar by placing the radiolabeled substance on top of the agar, allowing diffusion to occur, and removing the gel and sectioning it. From the concentration at different depths, the diffusion coefficients can be determined. Sucrose diffuses into brain at a rate of 3.0×10^{-6} cm^2/second. This is less than the rate of sucrose diffusion in agar (7.0×10^{-6} cm^2/second). Large molecules, such as polyethylene glycol, diffuse at a slower rate. Very large substances, such as dextran (MW 70,000) enter the brain to a very limited extent.

Autoradiography and computer imaging methods have been used to calculate diffusion coefficients. In studies carried out with the direct injection of a radiolabeled substance into brain, the rate of diffusion in a radial direction was determined (Rosenberg et al., 1988).

Substances injected directly into brain tissue are cleared at a rate dependent on multiple factors. An equation describing the exit of substances from brain after injection into the caudate has been developed (Cserr et al., 1978).

$$N_b = N_i e^{-kt} \tag{4-42}$$

Where N_b (dpm) is the total radioactivity remaining in brain at the end of the experiment, N_i (dpm) is the total amount injected into brain, and k is the first-order rate constant for total isotope efflux from brain (second^{-1}).

When substances of different molecular weights are injected into rat caudate, they leave at the same rate, indicating that they are removed by bulk flow rather than diffusion. The reason for this is that the rate of diffusion is dependent on the molecular weight and concentration, whereas bulk flow is driven by hydrostatic and osmotic pressure and is independent of molecular weight.

Diffusion from a point source has been calculated (Nicholson, 1985) and requires analysis of diffusion in two dimensions. Micropipettes have been used to measure the rate of diffusion and the extracellular space after microinjection.

4.12 MODELS AND MEASUREMENTS

The existence of a number of methods to measure capillary transport, blood flow, and intracerebral fluid flow indicates the lack of a best method to solve each of these problems. The accuracy of the numbers generated by the various equations depends on the appropriateness of the underlying mathematical model. For example, use of the brain uptake index to measure transport of sucrose, which is very slowly transported, will give an erroneous value. A better approach would be to use the intravenous methods that allow for the slow uptake during multiple passes of the blood through the brain. Similarly, if the information desired is simply whether the blood–brain barrier is open, the use of a dye with gross or microscopic visualization is the appropriate method.

Use of models to analyze biological data has provided the framework for comparisons based on quantitative measurements. The models are mathematical constructs with inherent assumptions. Testing of the models and the underlying assumptions require performing experiments under varying conditions that explore the outer limits of the assumptions. Once the boundaries within which the model applies are understood, the correct interpretation of the results is possible.

In performing transport studies, the first step is to choose the method best suited to the conditions of the experiment. The next step is to be sure that the assumptions underlying the method are met: Are there pathological changes that will deviate too far from the assumptions? Finally, the measurements need to be made in a reproducible manner without excessive scatter in the data, preventing proper statistical analysis. This can be done by careful attention to the variables in the experiment, such as species, anesthesia, feeding time, injection method, and injection solution. Variability in the data that is inherent in the experiment will then determine the number of experiments needed to reach statistical significance.

There are several methods of statistical analysis that are generally accepted, depending on the type of experimental data available. In the case of a simple comparison of two groups, one treated with an agent to be tested and the other untreated, the best test is Student's t-test. If the data fall out of the bell-shaped curve distribution, a nonparametric test must be used.

These tests are based on the rank-order of the results rather than the actual number. Biological data frequently require nonparametric analysis, and the Wilcoxon modification of the t-test is a useful measure of statistical significance (Dixon and Massey, 1969).

Often it is necessary to compare several treatments. In that case, it is possible that one of the t-tests could be significant on a random basis rather than because the results were significant. Therefore, a test for multiple comparisons must be done that takes into account the number of single comparisons. The test most commonly used is the one-way analysis of variance. For example, the results of several doses of a drug can be compared to the results with an untreated group. If another variable is introduced, such as the sex of the animal along with the dose effect, the test is a two-way analysis of variance. The groups are compared individually to a composite of all the values; when one or more groups stand out from the rest, the F value is high, and the likelihood of this being a random event is very low. When a high F value is obtained in the one-way analysis of variance, indicating that the differences are statistically significant, individual groups then can be compared for statistical significance with the control group and with each other. The greater the number of comparisons, the more stringent the statistical requirements for significance.

A difficult problem arises when within a large dataset several values stand far outside the majority of the numbers. Outliers, as these values are called, occur in biological experiments for a number of reasons. Including them in the statistical results removes the possibility of reaching statistical significance because of the wide standard deviation (SD). Increasing the number of experiments is both costly and wasteful of animals. Statistical methods have been developed to analyze data systematically, locate the outliers, and remove them from the analysis. One method is the Box plot, named after the person who devised the test. The median rather than the mean is used to define the dataset, and the spread within the majority of the data points is determined. Outliers are systematically removed from the cluster of points around the median. Both the control and experimental groups are treated similarly so that any bias is eliminated (Koopmans, 1987).

A hypothesis also can be tested by relating one variable to another to determine their correlaton. Linear regression determines how closely the data fit a straight line; the closer the correlation coefficient is to 1, the more significant the relationship. Linear relationships are important in biological data when two variables, such as carbon dioxide level and cerebral blood flow, can be varied over a range of numbers.

The likelihood of a relationship being present rather than a random occurrence is expressed as the significance level. In biological experiments, significance generally is taken as a probability of this being a random event of less than 0.05 (5 percent). When designing experiments, it is important to determine the number of experiments needed to achieve statistical significance. The SD of a series of pilot experiments is very useful for these estimates. Increasing the number of experiments improves the reliability.

However, this needs to be balanced with the need to use as few animals as possible. Therefore, careful planning of a series of experiments, often in conjunction with a statistician from the onset, is best.

REFERENCES

Betz, A. L., Iannotti, F.: Simultaneous determination of regional cerebral blood flow and blood–brain glucose transport kinetics in the gerbil. J. Cereb. Blood Flow Metab. 3:193–199, 1983.

Blasberg, R. G., Patlak, C. S., Fenstermacher, J. D.: Selecton of experimental conditions for the accurate determination of blood–brain transfer constants from single-time experiments: A theoretical analysis. J. Cereb. Blood Flow Metab. 3:215–225, 1983.

Bradbury, M. W., Patlak, C. S., Oldendorf, W. H.: Analysis of brain uptake and loss of radiotracers after intracarotid injection. Am. J. Physiol. 229:1110–1115, 1975.

Crone, C.: Facilitated transfer of glucose from blood into brain tissue. J. Physiol. 181:103–113, 1965.

Cserr, H. F., Berman, B. J.: Iodide and thiocyanate efflux from brain following injection into rat caudate nucleus. Am. J. Physiol. 235:331–337, 1978.

Daniel, P. M., Pratt, O. E., Wilson, P. A.: The transport of L-leucine into the brain of the rat in vivo: Saturable and non-saturable components of influx. Proc. R. Soc. Lond. [Biol.] 196:333–346, 1977.

Davson, H.: *Physiology of the Cerebrospinal Fluid.* Boston: Little, Brown and Co., 1967.

Davson, H., Segal, M. B.: The effects of some inhibitors and accelerators of sodium transport in the turnover of ^{22}Na in the cerebrospinal fluid and the brain. J. Physiol. 209:131–153, 1970.

Davson, H., Welch, K.: The permeation of several materials into the fluids of the rabbit's brain. J. Physiol. (London) 218:337–351, 1971.

Dixon, W. J., Massey, F. J., Jr.: *Introduction to Statistical Analysis.* New York: McGraw-Hill, 1969.

Katzman, R., Graziani, L., Ginsburg, S.: Cation exchange in blood, brain and CSF. Prog. Brain Res. 29:283–296, 1968.

Kety, S. S., Schmidt, C. F.: The nitrous oxide method for the quantitative determination of cerebral blood flow in man: Theory, procedure and normal values. J. Clin. Invest. 27:476–483, 1948.

Koopmans, L. H.: *An Introduction to Contemporary Statistics.* 2d ed. Boston: Duxbury Press, 1987.

Nicholson, C.: Diffusion from an injected volume of a substance in brain tissue with arbitrary volume fraction and tortuosity. Brain Res. 333:325–329, 1985.

Ohno, K., Pettigrew, K. D., Rapoport, S. I.: Lower limits of cerebrovascular permeability to nonelectrolytes in the conscious rat. Am. J. Physiol. 235:299–307, 1978.

Oldendorf, W. H.: Measurement of brain uptake of radiolabeled substances using a tritiated water internal standard. Brain Res. 24:372–376, 1970.

Oldendorf, W. H.: Clearance of radiolabeled substances by brain after arterial injection using a diffusible internal standard. In *Research Methods in Neurochemistry.* Marks, N., Rodnight, R., eds. New York: Plenum Press, 1981.

Pappenheimer, J. R., Heisey, S. R., Jordon, E. F., Downer, J. dec.: Perfusion of the cerebral ventricular system in unanesthetized goats. Am. J. Physiol. 203:763–774, 1962.

Pardridge, W. M.: Brain metabolism: A perspective from the blood–brain barrier. Physiol. Rev. 63:1481–1535, 1983.

Patlak, C. S., Fenstermacher, J. D.: Measurements of dog blood–brain transfer constants by ventriculocisternal perfusion. Am. J. Physiol. 229:877–884, 1975.

Raichle, M. E., Eichling, J. O., Grubb, R. L., Jr.: Brain permeability of water. Arch. Neurol. 30:319–321, 1974.

Raichle, M. E., Eichling, J. O., Straatmann, M. G., Welch, M. J., Larson, K. B., Ter Pogossian, M. M.: Blood–brain barrier permeability of ^{11}C-labeled alcohols and^{15}O-labeled water. Am. J. Physiol. 230:543–552, 1976.

Rall, D. P., Oppelt, W. W., Patlak, C. S.: Extracellular space of brain as determined by diffusion of inulin from the ventricular system. Life Sci. 1:43–48, 1962.

Rapoport, S. I., Ohno, K., Pettigrew, K. D.: Drug entry into the brain. Brain Res. 172:354–359, 1979.

Rosenberg, G. A., Barrett, J., Estrada, E., Brayer, J., Kyner, W. T.: Selective effect of mannitol-induced hyperosmolality on brain interstitial fluid and water content in white matter. Metab. Brain Dis. 3:217–227, 1988.

Rosenberg, G. A., Kyner, W. T., Estrada, E.: Bulk flow of brain interstitial fluid under normal and hyperosmolar conditions. Am. J. Physiol. 238:42–49, 1980.

Sakurada, O., Kennedy, C., Jehle, J., Brown, J. D., Carbin, G. L., Sokoloff, L.: Measurement of local cerebral blood flow with iodo [^{14}C] antipyrine. Am. J. Physiol. 234:59–66, 1978.

Smith, Q. R.: Methods to determine blood–brain barrier permeability and transport. Neuromethods 1:389–418, 1985.

Symon, L., Pasztor, E., Branston, N. M.: The distribution and density of reduced cerebral blood flow following acute middle cerebral artery occlusion: An experimental study by the technique of hydrogen clearance in baboons. Stroke 5:355–364, 1974.

Takasato, Y., Rapoport, S. I., Smith, Q. R.: An in situ brain perfusion technique to study cerebrovascular transport in the rat. Am. J. Physiol. 247:H484–H493, 1984.

Uyama, O., Okamura, N., Yanase, M., Narita, M., Kawabata, K., Sugita, M.: Quantitative evaluation of vascular permeability in the gerbil brain after transient ischemia using Evans blue fluorescence. J. Cereb. Blood Flow Metab. 8:282–284, 1988.

5

Radioisotopes in Metabolic Studies

5.1 INTRODUCTION

There are several methods for measurement of anatomical detail and physiological function in patients. Excellent anatomical detail is shown by CT and MRI. The imaging methods have had an immediate impact on patient care and have made obsolete pneumoencephalography and conventional nuclear brain scanning and reduced the need for EEG and ultrasound studies of brain. They have refined the indications for angiography and increased the ratio of abnormal studies to normal ones. Of less immediate impact but of greater future impact on the study of brain function are the minimally invasive method, PET, and the noninvasive method, NMR spectroscopy (Table 5–1).

The introduction of PET scanning into clinical investigations was made possible by advances in several areas. These include the development of autoradiographic methods to measure CBF and glucose use, the integration of the laws of decay of positron-labeled radioisotopes into isotope selection, and the development of radiochemical techniques capable of incorporating positron-labeled elements into physiological markers. An additional factor was the rapid advancements in the computer algorithms used to reconstruct CT scan images. The concepts of autoradiography and PET are similar, the major differences being the method of radioactivity detection. Autoradiograms are formed on x-ray film from thin slices of postmortem tissue while positrons are detected in vivo with sensors that detect radioactivity. Furthermore, ^{14}C-labeled substrates that were developed for autoradiography and first used to measure regional brain metabolism and receptor binding have been labeled with positrons for use in PET studies.

Autoradiography gives a detailed map of the substance under analysis in a slice of brain tissue and has been used successfully to study glucose me-

Table 5–1. Clinical Methods to Image Brain and Measure Metabolism

Modality	Advantages
Computed tomography (CT)	Visualize brain structures, ventricular enlargement, and atrophy
Magnetic resonance imaging (MRI)	Improved anatomical detail without bone artifact and excellent gray–white differentiation
Positron emission tomography (PET)	Rapid, sensitive method to measure glucose metabolism, blood flow, blood volume, and receptors
Magnetic resonance spectroscopy (MRS)	In vivo metabolic studies with ^{31}P, ^{1}H, ^{19}F, and ^{13}C

tabolism, CBF, interstitial fluid movement, blood–brain barrier transport, and receptor binding. Although autoradiograms provide excellent spatial resolution for one point in time, temporal information is lacking because of the need to remove the brain. PET uses similar substrates to those used in autoradiography with the added advantage of allowing repeated measurements in the same subject. The ability to make several measurements over time is very useful for studying the evolution of a disease process, such as the changes in metabolism that are seen in patients with seizures. Therefore, PET scanning has provided unique information on brain metabolism of glucose and oxygen, on blood flow, and on receptors in normal and pathological conditions (Phelps and Mazziotta, 1985; Raichle, 1986).

The third technological advance for analysis of brain function is NMR spectroscopy. This chapter describes the use of autoradiography and PET in studies of brain metabolism, and Chapter 6 describes the use of NMR.

5.2 AUTORADIOGRAPHY

The production of an autoradiographic image is possible because radioactive substances emit energized particles that expose x-ray films. The most commonly used radioactive substances are the beta-ray emitters, ^{14}C and ^{3}H, and the higher energy gamma rays. Beta rays are low-energy particles with half-lives of 5,580 years for ^{14}C and 12.5 years for ^{3}H, whereas gamma rays are more energetic, with shorter half-lives. Radioactive isotopes generally are detected in tracer quantities by liquid scintillation counting. Liquid scintillation counters have sensing devices that are activated by photons of light (Figure 5–1). Energy from a low-energy beta particle excites special light-sensitive molecules in solution, which in turn release photons. The photons are counted by a light-sensitive detection device, and the number of photons sensed is proportional to the radioactivity present. For scintillation counting, the excited molecules are in solution. However, when the excited medium is an x-ray film, location and quantification of the radioactivity in the tissue exposed to the film are possible. In autoradiography, the tissue containing the isotopically labeled substance of interest is placed in contact with an x-

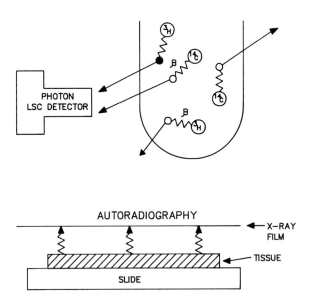

AUTORADIOGRAPHY

Figure 5–1. Methods for detection of radioactivity. Top. Liquid scintillation count-ing is the release of photons (straight arrows) after excitation by beta rays (jagged arrows) from ^{14}C or ^{3}H molecules. The photons are counted by a light-sensitive device (LSC). Bottom. Autoradiography involves exposure of x-ray film to a source of radioactivity in tissue, generally on a slide.

ray film or a slide containing a gel sensitive to radioactivity (Figure 5–1). The regions exposed to the radioactivity show up as darkened areas when the film is developed. The concentration of the radiolabeled material in the tissue is quantitated by exposing the film at the same time to a set of stan-dards with increasing amounts of isotope. Quantitative autoradiography is done by comparing film densities of standards with a known radioactive content to those of the tissue regions exposed at the same time. Autoradio-grams made with ^{3}H have better spatial resolution than do those made with ^{14}C because of the lower energy and shorter path length of the ^{3}H beta ray. Quantitation of ^{3}H is more difficult because of self-absorption of the low-energy ^{3}H particle by the tissue. Under optimal conditions, the resolution of ^{14}C-autoradiography is approximately 0.1 mm.

The spectroscopic and autoradiographic methods of liquid scintillation, x-ray exposure, and NMR are a measure of the amount of substrate rather than its concentration. A small volume of a highly concentrated solution will give the same number of counts or x-ray intensity as a larger amount of a less concentrated solution (Figure 5–2). Therefore, it is essential to know the volume of the solution or the area of the autoradiogram before a calculation of concentration can be made. This becomes important in in vivo NMR spectroscopy where the volume is uncertain, making the quantification of the spectra difficult.

Preparation of an autoradiogram requires injection of an animal with the

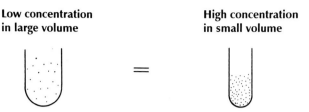

Low concentration
in large volume

High concentration
in small volume

Figure 5–2. Spectroscopic and autoradiographic methods, including liquid scintillation counting, autoradiograms, PET, and NMR, measure total amount of a substance. In order to obtain concentration, the volume must be known.

isotopically labeled substance. After a given time, the animal is killed, and the brain is removed and frozen. Frozen tissue containing the isotope is sectioned on a cryostat and placed on a slide. The sectioned tissue is exposed to an x-ray film. A set of ^{14}C-standards with a known amount of radioactivity is exposed along with the tissue sections. The film is developed after a given time period that depends on the isotope used, the type of x-ray film, and the concentration of the isotope. A given area of the exposed film is analyzed by a densitometer and converted to concentration of ^{14}C in dpm/mg by a computer that has an optical density curve established from the same area of a set of standards (Figure 5–3).

Several types of densitometers are available, including a microdensitometer that digitizes the film point by point over small distances, a rotating drum digitizer that rapidly reads entire x-rays, and a videocamera connected to an imaging computer that is most widely used because it is both rapid and convenient. The video image is digitized and enhanced by the computer. The isotope concentration is determined from the standards developed on

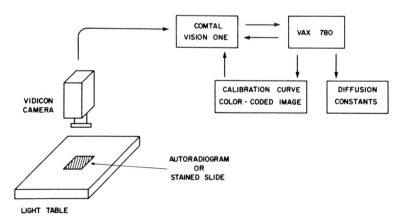

Figure 5–3. Image processor for analysis of x-ray films. Television camera (vidicon) reads images. An image processor (COMTAL) assigns optical densities to each point in a 512 × 512 matrix. Optical densities compared with standard curve in a computer (VAX) and final image pseudocolored according to concentration of the isotope.

the film. The final image can be color-coded for display on the videomonitor (Goochee et al., 1980).

Values for autoradiograms can be expressed in disintegrations per minute (dpm) per amount of tissue. From a set of known standards, the optical densities read by the imaging device are converted to dpm/g with a curve fitting procedure. The optical density value of the x-ray film exposed to the tissue sample is interpolated to the concentration of isotope in the tissue. Colors are added to create a pseudocolor map to enhance the visual display, but the basic information is contained in the original black and white image.

Differentiation of one brain region from another is difficult from auto-radiograms, since distinctions between gray and white matter may not be evident, and the anatomy may be distorted by a pathological process. Staining the contiguous slide section aids in identifying regions of interest, but distortion of tissue sections may occur with sectioning. After the x-ray image is obtained, the same tissue section that was exposed to the x-ray film is stained. A computer image processor is used to superimpose and align the x-ray and stained tissue image (Figure 5–4).

In some experiments, it is desirable to have simultaneous use of two different isotopes for autoradiograms. Useful information is obtainable with the use of two isotopes, as in the simultaneous measurement of blood flow and glucose metabolism. One method of measuring both ^{14}C and ^{3}H in the same piece of tissue is to use a much higher dose of ^{3}H than ^{14}C. The tissue is initially exposed for 5 weeks to a film (MR-1, Kodak Corp.) that mainly is sensitive to ^{14}C. A second film sensitive to both ^{14}C and ^{3}H (Ultrofilm, LKB Products) is exposed for 2 weeks. The ^{14}C from the first film is subtracted from the ^{14}C and ^{3}H in the second, and with correction for excessive ^{3}H absorption by white matter, the amount of both tracers in the tissue can be calculated (Juhler and Diemer, 1987).

Analysis of receptor binding has become possible with the development of labeled receptor ligands. In vitro receptor binding is done in specially prepared tissue sections. The sectioned tissue is placed in baths with the isotopically labeled ligand. The label adheres to the receptor site and subsequently can be detected after exposure to x-ray film for several weeks. It is necessary to determine the nonspecific binding by incubating another tissue section in a bath with both the labeled ligand and a larger quantity of unlabeled or cold ligand, which will block the label from the receptor and allow measurement of nonspecific binding.

Autoradiograms have been made from several ^{3}H and ^{14}C-labeled compounds and have been used to measure cerebral function, such as glucose metabolism (Sokoloff et al., 1977; Kennedy et al., 1976), CBF (Reivich et al., 1969; Sakurada et al., 1978), blood–brain barrier permeability (Blasberg et al., 1983), ISF movement (Rosenberg et al., 1988), precursor-transmitter accumulation, and receptor binding (Kuhar et al., 1986) (Table 5–2). The in vitro autoradiographic studies have prepared the way for in vivo isotopic analysis with positron-labeled molecules by PET.

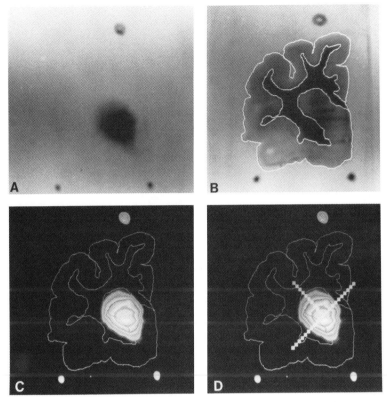

Figure 5–4. Example of computer analysis. Animal injected with radiolabeled substance into caudate for diffusion measurements. A. The x-ray image of ^{14}C-sucrose. Note that anatomical detail is lacking. The three dots are for alignment with slide. B. Section (20 μm) stained for myelin (dark region) is entered into computer, and the white matter (dark) is outlined to separate it from cortex and caudate (light). C. Color-coded x-ray image and superimposed computer outline to show injection into caudate. D. Computer-generated squares used to measure optical density for diffusion calculations. (From Rosenberg et al., 1988)

Table 5–2. ^{14}C-Labeled Compounds Used in Autoradiography

^{14}C-Labeled Substrate	Function Studied	Reference
Deoxyglucose	Glucose metabolism	Sokoloff et al., 1977
Aminoisobutyric acid	Blood–brain barrier	Blasberg et. al., 1983
Iodoantipyrine	Cerebral blood flow	Sakurada et. al., 1978
Extracellular markers (sucrose and polyethylene glycol)	Interstitial fluid transport	Rosenberg et. al., 1988
Receptor ligands	Glutamate, dopamine receptors, etc.	Kuhar, 1986

5.3 POSITRON EMISSION TOMOGRAPHY

Positrons are positively charged particles emitted from an unstable nucleus. When a positron and electron collide, they are annihilated and two gamma rays are formed that are at a 180° angle to each other (Phelps et al., 1975). The PET scanner has an array of detectors arranged in a circle. An event is recorded when detectors at 180° to each other are simultaneously activated. A large array of opposing radiation detectors allows localization of the point source of positron emission. The detection of two simultaneous events is recorded for multiple lines of coincidence, and the data are reconstructed analogously to CT scanning. The principles used for data analysis and image reconstruction are similar for CT, MRI, and PET. The major benefits of PET scanning are that it allows location of the point source in three dimensions and that very small amounts of tracer can be detected.

The positron-emitting atoms commonly used for labeling for PET studies are ^{15}O, ^{13}N, ^{11}C, and ^{18}F, with half-lives of 2, 10, 20, and 110 minutes, respectively. These compounds are given in from 5 to 100 millicurie (mCi) doses depending on the compound labeled and the organ to be studied. The total radiation dose to the patient is from 1 to 2 rads, with a maximum permissible dose of 5 rads. Repeated studies with certain compounds can, therefore, lead to appreciable radiation exposure (Raichle, 1983).

PET was developed as a tomographic extension of nuclear isotope scanning and has been applied to studies of metabolism and blood flow in humans (Phelps et al., 1979; Kuhl, 1984). The short-lived positrons are produced by a cyclotron and immediately attached to the compound of interest. The positron-containing compounds or, in some cases, the atoms themselves are injected into the experimental subjects. The cyclotron is located next to the scanner. PET scanners and cyclotrons are expensive to operate and require a team of physicists, chemists, and physicians. High costs for equipment and personnel have limited these instruments to a few large centers.

Gamma-emitting atoms have been studied by single photon emission computed tomography (SPECT). SPECT instruments are less expensive and easier to operate than PET scanners, but gamma-emitting isotopes of carbon, nitrogen, or oxygen are unavailable, and it is difficult to trace metabolic pathways with SPECT. On the other hand, iodoamphetamine-labeled with ^{123}I has been used to measure CBF with SPECT, and labeled compounds that bind to brain receptors have been developed.

PET, like autoradiography, shows regional substrate use (Table 5–3). Instead of a beta or gamma emitter, a positron emitter is used. For example, glucose metabolism is measured with 2-deoxy-2-[^{18}F]fluro-D-glucose (FDG), which is phosphorylated on entry into brain cells and trapped as the phosphorylated compound (Huang et al., 1980). Since little of the tracer is metabolized in the first few minutes, transport into brain cells can be measured. Some of the originally injected tracer remains in blood and extracellular fluid during this short time period, making corrections for regional blood volume necessary. Generally, a 30–40 minute delay after injection is necessary for

Table 5–3. Positron Radionuclides Incorporated into Molecules of Biological Importance

Radionuclide	Compound	Function Tested
Fluorine-18	Deoxyglucose	Glucose metabolism
	Methylspiperone	Dopamine receptors
	Fluoro-L-dopa	Dopa metabolism
Carbon-11	Carbon monoxide	Blood volume
	Dimethyloxazalidinedione (DMO)	Brain pH
	Glucose	Glucose transport
	Diazepam	Valium receptors
	Carfentanil	Opiate receptors
Oxygen-15	Oxygen	Oxygen extraction
	Carbon dioxide	Blood flow
	Water	Blood flow
Nitrogen-13	Amino acids	Protein synthesis
Rubidium-82	Rubidium chloride	Blood–brain barrier

complete phosphorylation of the tracer, and during this time, some metabolism by phosphatase may occur. The problem with use of an analog are the long measurement time, the large radiation dose, particularly with ^{18}F (110 minute half-life compared to 20 minutes for ^{11}C), and the potential toxicity from compounds that interfere with glucose metabolism.

Several methods have been used to measure CBF and oxygen metabolism with PET. The ^{15}O steady-state inhalation model provides measurements of regional cerebral blood flow (rCBF), oxygen extraction ratio (rOER), and oxygen use ($rCMRO_2$) (Jones et al., 1976; Frackowiak et al., 1980). The basis of the technique involves the continuous inhalation of tracer amounts of $C^{15}O_2$. In the lungs, the CO_2 is converted to ^{15}O-water. After 10 minutes, a steady-state is reached, with the rate of delivery to the brain balanced by the washout of the tracer into the venous circulation. rCBF is related to the arterial (C_a) and tissue (C_i) concentrations of ^{15}O-water by the relationship

$$rCBF = \tau/[(C_a/C_i) - 1] \qquad (5-1)$$

where τ is a correction factor to account for loss from decay (Leenders et al., 1984). The rOER is measured by the inhalation of $^{15}O_2$ with corrections for recirculation of labeled water. From the blood flow and oxygen extraction, the $rCMRO_2$ can be determined.

$$CMRO_2 = CBF \times [O_2]_{arterial} \times OER \qquad (5-2)$$

Errors in the use of these equations occur because the extraction of H_2O is less than 100 percent and because of variability of cerebral blood volume, which needs to be calculated from ^{11}CO. Current models of rCBF and rOER measurement incorporate terms to correct for these factors (Lammertsma and Jones, 1983). Measurements of rCBF and rOER with the steady-state continuous inhalation method require 1.5–2 hours. Patient cooperation is essential for these long studies.

Another method to measure CBF by PET besides inhalation of ^{15}O-labeled CO_2 (Frackowiak et al., 1980) is the injection of ^{15}O-water (Huang et al., 1983; Raichle et al., 1983). ^{15}O is well suited to blood flow measurements because it has a short half-life and can, therefore, be used for repeated measurements without producing too great a radiation exposure. Measurement of cerebral blood flow with ^{15}O-water is based on the Kety approach to describing the exchange of an inert gas between blood and tissue. ^{15}O-water is injected intravenously, and arterial samples are collected over several minutes while the ^{15}O is detected in the brain. The main problem with the use of ^{15}O-water is that it is not freely diffusable across the capillary. The diffusion rate for water is slower than for a freely diffusable substance (Raichle et al., 1974). Blood flows estimated with water are underestimated (Eckman et al., 1975). The advantage of the use of ^{15}O-water is that it has a short half-life with low radiation exposure from a single study, making multiple studies possible in a single subject (Herscovitch et al., 1983).

The extent of the diffusion limitation with water has been studied with a more readily diffusable substance, ^{11}C-butanol, which is an alcohol that easily crosses the blood–brain barrier (Raichle et al., 1976; Sage et al., 1981). Compared to water, it is more completely extracted. The amount of butanol and water extracted by the brain differs; the difference in the amount of each isotope extracted by the brain provides a means to calculate the permeability of the capillary to water (Herscovitch et al., 1987). For low flow rates, labeled water gives an accurate estimation of the blood flow; however, at high flow rates greater than 120 ml/minute/100 g, the estimation becomes inaccurate (Figure 5–5). From these measurements in humans, the permeability surface area (PS) for human cortex is estimated to be 127 ml/minute/ 100 g. The higher the rate of blood flow, the greater the PS product. Since the permeability is probably similar for all capillaries, the regional differences are due to the high capillary density in some regions compared to others.

Although ^{11}C-butanol is a better compound to use to measure CBF, it has several disadvantages that limit its usefulness. The longer half-life of ^{11}C results in a slow decay of the radioactivity, which interferes with subsequent isotopic studies and limits the number of times blood flow can be measured. For this reason, the ^{15}O-labeled compounds have been used more frequently to measure CBF.

CBF follows function. During mental or physical activity, areas of the brain involved in that activity increase their blood flow. The increases and decreases in activity occur in a very short time frame, but prolonged stimulus can maintain that activity. In order to use PET scanning to study motor, sensory, or mental actions, measurement of either deoxyglucose use or blood flow has been done. The former requires 20–40 minutes to complete a study, whereas the latter study can be performed in under 1 minute.

Repeated measurements of cerebral blood flow with ^{15}O-water in normal

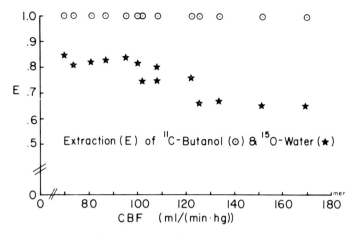

Figure 5–5. Fraction of ^{11}C-butanol and ^{15}O-H$_2$O extracted during a single cerebral passage, plotted as a function of blood flow. In contrast to the declining extraction (E) of ^{15}O-H$_2$O observed with increasing blood flow, in no case was an unextracted fraction observed with ^{11}C-butanol. (From Herscovitch et al., 1987)

subjects have been used to follow complex cognitive processes (Peterson et al., 1988; Posner et al., 1988). Use of PET in conjunction with cognitive testing allows localization of the neural system involved in cognitive operations in the brain. These studies show that the brain has localized centers for mental operations. Activation of these processes requires coordination of multiple brain areas, with timing being important. The elementary operations that are part of a cognitive analysis are localized to specific regions, whereas a single complex task involves multiple brain areas. The tasks involved in forming visual images were studied in normal subjects by breaking down the task into its multiple components. Visual recognition was tested by presenting letters to the subject while cerebral blood flow was measured. A control state was first recorded and then subtracted from the stimulus state. By this means, variability among subjects could be reduced as subjects became their own controls, and fewer subjects could be studied to obtain meaningful data in spite of the wide subject-to-subject variability. Visual tasks were entirely coded within the occipital lobe. Two activated areas from letter-matching tasks were identified along the calcarine fissure of the left and right primary visual cortex and three in the left and right lateral regions. When the subjects were asked to associate an activity with an image (pound with hammer), the subtracted scans showed activation of the anterior left frontal lobe. These studies demonstrated that word reading is an automatic activity that does not require participation of the visual–spatial system in the parietal lobe. Thus, PET scanning studies provide a powerful method to analyze cognitive function.

In addition to the studies of blood flow and metabolism with labeled water, oxygen, and deoxyglucose, other labeled molecules have been used to analyze blood–brain barrier integrity, protein synthesis, and receptor binding.

The integrity of the blood–brain barrier has been analyzed with rubidium-82, a potassium analog that normally is excluded from the brain (Brooks et al., 1984). Patients with cerebral infarctions and brain tumors have an increased uptake of the tracer because of damage to their blood–brain barriers.

Imaging of brain neurotransmitter receptors with positron-labeled receptor binding molecules has been used to study patients with parkinsonism, schizophrenia, and epilepsy. Engel et al. (1982) have used PET scanning to study glucose metabolism in patients with temporal lobe epilepsy. Interictally, the abnormal temporal lobe is hypometabolic, and it becomes hypermetabolic during a seizure. The localization of the abnormal tissue for surgical removal is aided by PET scanning (Figure 5–6). The dopamine D2 receptor has been imaged in humans with the receptor ligand, ^{11}C-N-methylspiperone (Wagner et al., 1983). Normally, the ligand binds specifically to the dopamine receptors in the caudate (Figure 5–7). The potential use-

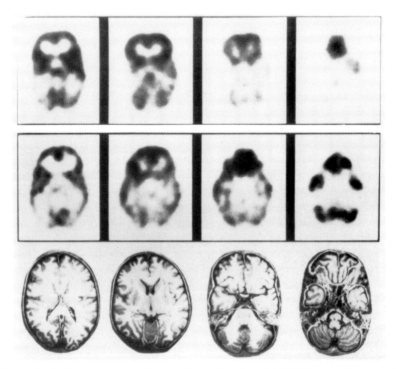

Figure 5–6. Four representative sections of an interictal FDG scan from a patient with partial complex seizures (top) show a zone of relative hypometabolism in the left temporal lobe. The hypometabolic area can be appreciated on all planes through the temporal lobe. Similar sections from a scan taken from a volunteer subject (middle) are normal. Some asymmetry of temporal lobe metabolism is present in the far left section, but since this was seen only in one plane it may reflect head rotation and cannot be considered abnormal. Photographs (bottom) show anatomical features included in planes of section more clearly. (From Engel et al., 1982)

fulness of receptor studies is demonstrated by a study by Wong et al. (1984) that showed that aging caused a fall in the number of dopamine D2 receptors in the caudate.

PET has been used to study other receptors, including those to opiates. Opiate receptors are found in high concentration in several brain regions, including the medial thalamus, amygdala, and spinal cord (Pert and Snyder, 1973). Imaging of opiate receptors was accomplished with the morphine-like drug, 4-carbomethoxyfentanyl (carfentanil) (Frost et al., 1985). The opiate antagonist, naloxon, inhibited carfentanil binding (Figure 5–8).

Patients with the dominantly inherited movement disorder, Huntington's chorea, have a reduction of glucose metabolism in the caudate (Kuhl et al., 1982). Some asymptomatic carriers also have shown hypometabolism of the caudate before structural changes (Berent et al., 1988). The overlapping of the data points between affected individuals who will develop the disease and normal relatives is still too great for prediction of those with the Huntington gene. Patients with olivopontocerebellar atrophy have reduced glucose metabolism in the cerebellum and brainstem (Kluin et al., 1988).

Thus, PET scanning has provided important new information on the pathophysiology of several neurological illnesses. In addition to the insights it offers in disease states, it should be able to provide information on the organization of the brain in normal individuals. The high cost and technical requirements of the instrument will, however, limit its usefulness in the near future to a few research centers.

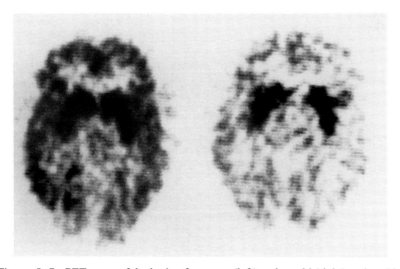

Figure 5–7. PET scans of the brain of a young (left) and an old (right) male subject. Dopamine D_2 receptors are labeled with ^{11}C-3-N-methylspiperone. The dark areas in the center are the basal ganglia. Reduced uptake is seen in the elderly subject. (From Wong et al., 1984)

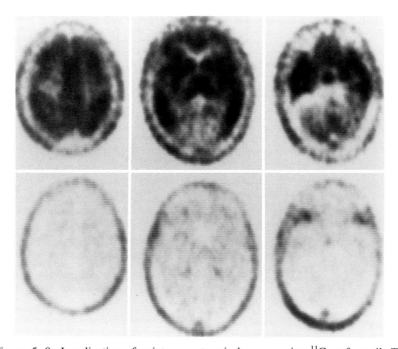

Figure 5–8. Localization of opiate receptors in humans using ^{11}C-carfentanil. The images in the top row were obtained using the Neuro ECAT 30–60 minute after intravenous administration of 25 mCi ^{11}C-carfentanil, 80 ng/kg. The three images were localized using x-ray CT at approximately 7.2, 4, and 0.8 cm above the canthomeatal line, respectively. Images in the bottom row were acquired at the same time following intravenous administration of the opiate antagonist naloxone, 1 mg/kg, and the same dose of ^{11}C-carfentanil used in the first study. The brightness of each image is normalized for the injected activity, the acquisition time, and radioactive decay. A preferential accumulation of activity is seen in areas known to contain high concentrations of opiate receptors, such as the thalamus, basal ganglia, pituitary gland, and cortex. Conversely, low activity is seen where opiate receptors exist in low concentrations, such as the occipital cortex, the postcentral gyrus, and the cerebellum. The images in the bottom row demonstrate the low level of nonreceptor binding in the brain and pituitary gland. Binding is not inhibited in the skull or venous sinuses. (From Frost et al., 1985)

REFERENCES

Berent, S., Giordani, B., Lehtinen, S., Markel, D., Penney, J. B., Buchtel, H. A., Starosta-Rubinstein, S., Hichwa, R., Young, A. B.: Positron emission tomographic scan investigation of Huntington's disease: Cerebral metabolic correlates of cognitive function. Ann. Neurol. 23:541–546, 1988.

Blasberg, R. G., Fenstermacher, J. D., Patlak, C. S.: Transport of alpha-aminoisobutyric acid across brain capillary and cellular membranes. J. Cereb. Flow Metab. 3:8–32, 1983.

Brooks, D. J., Beaney, R. P., Lammertsma, A. A., Leenders, K. L., et. al.: Quantitative measurement of blood–brain barrier permeability using [82]Rb and positron emission tomography. J. Cereb. Blood. Flow Metab. 4:535–545, 1984.

Eckman, W. W., Phair, R. D., Fenstermacher, J. D., Patlak, C. S., Kennedy, C., Sokoloff, L.: Permeability limitation in estimation of local brain blood flow with [^{14}C]antipyrine. Am. J. Physiol. 229:215–221, 1975.

Engel, J., Jr., Kuhl, D. E., Phelps, M. E., Mazziotta, J. C.: Interictal cerebral glucose metabolism in partial epilepsy and its relation to EEG changes. Ann. Neurol. 12:510–517, 1982.

Frackowiak, R. S. J., Lenzi, G. L., Jones, T., Heather, J. D.: Quantitative measurement of regional cerebral blood flow and oxygen metabolism in man using [15]O and positron emission tomography: Theory, procedure, and normal value. J. Comput. Assist. Tomogr. 4:727–736, 1980.

Frost, J. J., Wagner, H. N., Jr., Dannals, R. F., Ravert, H. T., Links, J. M., Wilson, A. A., Burns, H. D., Wong, D. F., McPherson, R. W., Rosenbaum, A. E., et. al.: Imaging opiate receptors in the human brain by positron tomography. J. Comput. Assist. Tomog. 9:231–236, 1985.

Goochee, C., Rasband, W., Sokoloff, L.: Computerized densitometry and color coding of [^{14}C] deoxyglucose autoradiographs. Ann. Neurol. 7:359–370, 1980.

Herscovitch, P., Markham, J., Raichle, M. E.: Brain blood flow measured with intravenous H_2[15]O. I. Theory and error analysis. J. Nucl. Med. 24:782–789, 1983.

Herscovitch, P., Raichle, M. E., Kilbourn, M. R., Welch, M. J.: Positron emission tomographic measurement of cerebral blood flow and permeability-surface area product of water using [^{15}O]water and [^{11}C]Butanol. J. Cereb. Blood Flow Metab. 7:527–542, 1987.

Huang, S. C., Carson, R. E., Hoffman, E. J., Carson, J., MacDonald, N., Barrio, J. R., Phelps, M. E.: Quantitative measurement of local cerebral blood flow in humans by positron computed tomography and [^{15}O]water. J. Cereb. Blood Flow Metab. 3:141–153, 1983.

Huang, S. C., Phelps, M. E., Hoffman, E. J., Sideris, K., Selin, C. J., Kuhl, D. E.: Noninvasive determination of local cerebral metabolic rate of glucose in man. Am. J. Physiol. 238:69–82, 1980.

Jones, T., Chesler, D. A., Ter-Pogossian, M. M.: The continuous inhalation of oxygen-15 for assessing regional oxygen extraction in the brain of man. Br. J. Radiol. 49:339–343, 1976.

Juhler, M., Diemer, N. H.: A method for ^{14}C and ^{3}H double-label autoradiography. J. Cereb. Blood Flow Metab. 7:572–577, 1987.

Kennedy, C., Des Rosiers, M. H., Sakurada, O., Shinohara, M., Reivich, M., Jehle, J. W., Sokoloff, L.: Metabolic mapping of the primary visual system of the monkey by means of the autoradiographic [^{14}C]deoxyglucose technique. Proc. Natl. Acad. Sci. USA 73:4230–4234, 1976.

Kluin, K. J., Gilman, S., Markel, D. S., Koeppe, R. A., Rosenthal, G., Junck, L.: Speech disorders in olivopontocerebellar atrophy correlate with positron emission tomography findings. Ann. Neurol. 23:547–554, 1988.

Kuhar, M. J., De Souza, E. B., Unnerstall, J. R.: Neurotransmitter receptor mapping by autoradiography and other methods. Annu. Rev. Neurosci. 9:27–59, 1986.

Kuhl, D. E.: Imaging local brain function with emission computed tomography. Radiology 150:625–631, 1984.

Kuhl, D. E., Phelps, M. E., Markham, C. H., Metter, E. J., Riege, W. H., Winter, J.: Cerebral metabolism and atrophy in Huntington's disease determined by [18]FDG and computed tomographic scan. Ann. Neurol. 12:425–434, 1982.

Lammertsma, A. A., Jones, T.: The correction for the presence of intravascular oxygen-15 in the steady-state technique for measuring regional oxygen extraction in the brain: I. Description of the method. J. Cereb. Blood Flow Metab. 3:416–424, 1983.

Leenders, K. L., Gibbs, J. M., Frackowiak, R. S. J., Lammertsma, A. A., Jones, T.: Positron emission tomography of the brain: New possibilities for the investigation of human cerebral pathophysiology. Prog. Neurobiol. 23:1–39, 1984.

Pert, C. B., Snyder, S. H.: Opiate receptor: Demonstration in nervous tissue. Science 179:1011–1014, 1973.

Peterson, S. E., Fox, P. T., Posner, M. I., Mintun, M., Raichle, M. E.: Positron emission tomographic studies of the cortical anatomy of single-word processing. Nature 331:585–589, 1988.

Phelps, M. E., Hoffman, E. J., Mullani, N. A., Ter Pogossian, M. M.: Application of annihilation coincidence detection to transaxial reconstruction tomography. J. Nucl. Med. 16:210–224, 1975.

Phelps, M. E., Huang, S. C., Hoffman, E. J., Selin, C., Sokoloff, L., Kuhl, D. E.: Tomographic measurement of local cerebral glucose metabolic rate in humans with (F-18)2-fluoro-2-deoxy-D-glucose: Validation of method. Ann. Neurol. 6:371–388, 1979.

Phelps, M. E., Mazziotta, J. C.: Positron emission tomography: Human brain function and biochemistry. Science 228:799–810, 1985.

Posner, M. I., Petersen, S. E., Fox, P. T., Raichle, M. E.: Localization of cognitive operations in the human brain. Science 240:1627–1631, 1988.

Raichle, M. E.: Positron emission tomography. Annu. Rev. Neurosci. 6:249–276, 1983.

Raichle, M. E.: Positron emission tomography with oxygen-15 radiopharmaceuticals. In *PET and NMR: New Perspectives in Neuroimaging and in Clinical Neurochemistry* Battistin, L., Gerstenbrand, F., eds. New York: Alan R. Liss, 1986:39–48.

Raichle, M. E., Eichling, J. O., Grubb, R. L., Jr.: Brain permeability of water. Arch. Neurol. 30:319–321, 1974.

Raichle, M. E., Eichling, J. O., Straatman, M. G., Welch, M. J., Larson, K. B., Ter-Pogossian, M. M.: Blood–brain barrier permeability of ^{11}C-labelled alcohols and ^{15}O-labelled water. Am. J. Physiol. 230:543–552, 1976.

Reivich, M., Jehle, J., Sokoloff, L., Kety, S. S.: Measurement of regional cerebral blood flow with antipyrine-^{14}C in awake cats. J. Appl. Physiol. 27:296–300, 1969.

Rosenberg, G. A., Barrett, J., Estrada, E., Brayer, J., Kyner, W. T.: Selective effect of mannitol-induced hyperosmolality on brain interstitial fluid and water content in white matter. Metab. Brain Dis. 3:217–227, 1988.

Sage, J. I., Van Uitert, R. L., Duffy, T. E.: Simultaneous measurement of cerebral blood flow and unidirectional movement of substances across the blood–brain barrier: Theory, method, and application to leucine. J. Neurochem. 36:1731–1738, 1981.

Sakurada, O., Kennedy, C., Jehle, J., Brown, J. D., Carbin, G. L., Sokoloff, L.:

Measurement of local cerebral blood flow with iodo [^{14}C] antipyrine. Am. J. Physiol. 234:59–66, 1978.

Sokoloff, L., Reivich, M., Kennedy, C., Des Rosiers, M. H., Patlak, C. S., Pettigrew, K. D., Sakurada, O., Shinohara, M.: The [^{14}C]deoxyglucose method for the measurement of local cerebral glucose utilization: Theory, procedure, and normal values in the conscious and anesthetized albino rat. J. Neurochem. 28:897–916, 1977.

Wagner, H. N., Jr., Burns, H. D., Dannals, R. F., Wong, D. F., Langstrom, B., Duelfer, T., Frost, J. J., Ravert, H. T., Links, J. M., Rosenbloom, S. B., Lukas, S. E., Kramer, A. V., Kuhar, M. J.: Imaging dopamine receptors in the human brain by positron tomography. Science 221:1264–1266, 1983.

Wong, D. F., Wagner, H. N., Jr., Dannals, R. F., Links, J. M., Frost, J. J., Ravert, H. T., Wilson, A. A., Rosenbaum, A. E., Gjedde, A., Douglass, K. H., et. al.: Effects of age on dopamine and serotonin receptors measured by positron tomography in the living human brain. Science 226:1393–1396, 1984.

6

Nuclear Magnetic Resonance
Spectroscopy

6.1 INTRODUCTION

Nuclear magnetic resonance (NMR) was described independently by Bloch and by Purcell in 1946, and they received the Nobel Prize in Physics in 1952 for their discovery. Initially, NMR was used exclusively to analyze chemical structure and follow chemical reactions. Lauterbur (1973) demonstrated the ability of NMR to form images. In the past 10 years, there have been major refinements in the design and operation of NMR spectrometers. Developments in magnet technology have led to higher fields, with improved homogeneity in large-bore magnets. Along with the application of computer methods from CT, it is now possible to use NMR in imaging and spectroscopy on living tissues.

Imaging and spectroscopy, although based on the same principles, are different applications on NMR. The rapid advances in computer algorithms for calculations used in CT were applied to the construction of images from NMR signals. Imaging uses gradient fields applied across the object to be imaged. This results in a slightly different magnetic field being experienced at different regions. The signals obtained are from the protons on water and vary according to the applied field. Therefore, they can be reconstructed to form an image. Spectroscopy of tissue, on the other hand, can be performed on signals from several different atoms within a given volume. Because NMR spectroscopy is a relatively insensitive method for atoms other than ^{1}H, the volume observed generally must be large or the collection time long.

Magnetic resonance imaging (MRI) is based on the magnetic properties of hydrogen atoms in water. High-resolution MRI instruments are available and have replaced CT scanners as the diagnostic method of choice in the brainstem, posterior fossa, and spinal cord. MRI has several advantages over CT scans: (1) it avoids the artifacts seen on CT in regions close to bone, (2) there is better differentiation of gray from white matter, and (3) flow phenomenon can be seen by MRI.

Another advantage of NMR over other methods, although still in its early stages of development, is spectroscopy, which provides a unique method for the in vivo study of metabolism, using atoms that are important for the study of biological processes, such as ^{13}C, ^{19}F, ^{23}Na, ^{31}P, and ^{1}H (Budinger and Lauterbur, 1984). Thus, in vivo noninvasive measurements of brain metabolism over time can be made with NMR spectroscopy (Prichard and Shulman, 1986).

6.2 BASIC CONCEPTS

6.2.1 Fundamental NMR Equation

The concepts of NMR are complex and require quantum mechanics for a full appreciation. The following discussion is greatly simplified and focused on those aspects necessary for an understanding of spectroscopy in biological systems. The explanations here are drawn heavily from several fundamental texts that contain excellent introductions to the subject (Abraham and Loftus, 1978; Shaw 1981; Gadian, 1982).

Nuclei with magnetic moments align themselves parallel to a magnetic field. Certain atoms possess the magnetic properties that make them detectable by NMR. Atoms have nuclear spin whose value depends on the mass number and the atomic number of the nucleus. Those nuclei with spins of 1/2, 3/2, 5/2, etc. will resonate when placed in an applied magnetic field. The resonant frequency will depend on the magnetogyric ratio, γ, which is a proportionality constant specific for each particular atom. The fundamental resonance condition for all NMR experiments is given by the equation

$$\nu_o = \gamma \, B_o/2\pi \qquad (6-1)$$

where, ν_o, is the frequency (Hz) at which a nucleus of a given magnetogyric ratio resonates when a magnetic field, B_o, is applied. The field or the frequency may be varied to obtain a spectrum.

The strength of a magnetic field is described in tesla (T) (1 T = 10 kilogauss). When nuclei with magnetic moments are excited with radiowaves of a specific frequency, they emit a signal of the same frequency as that applied. Atoms with magnetic moments can assume one of several discrete energy states when placed in a magnetic field. When an exciting field is applied, the atom undergoes transition from one energy state to another.

Energy levels in NMR are in the radiofrequency range of 10^7 Hz. Visible light is at a frequency of 10^{15}, and x-rays are 10^{17} (Figure 6–1). Therefore, the energy of the radiation needed for NMR studies is relatively low. Spec-

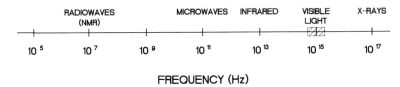

FREQUENCY (Hz)

Figure 6–1. Regions of the electromagnetic spectrum. The visible light region occupies a small band around 10^{15} Hz. NMR is in the radiowave energy level.

troscopy involves raising the energy level of a substance and recording its return to the unexcited state. Energy is absorbed and emitted in discrete packets. Increasing the energy state causes a transition to the higher level. Because magnetic moments of atoms are small, the amount of energy needed to raise their energy state is in the 10^5–10^7 Hz range. Excitation of electrons in the microwave range of 10^{11} Hz induces molecular rotation and heating. The NMR signal depends on the weak interaction of one nucleus with another; for example, ^1H near to a ^{13}C produces an interaction that slightly modifies the magnetic environment of the nucleus in the applied field.

The strength of the magnetic field can vary over a wide range from very low fields of 0.05 T (500 gauss) to high fields of 10 T (100,000 gauss). Imaging is possible with low-field permanent magnets. Magnets with field strength of 0.5 T have been found to be sufficient to detect hydrogen, and they have the advantage of being less expensive than supercooled magnets while still providing high-quality images. Superconducting, helium-cooled magnets are needed to produce the higher field strength for in vivo spectroscopy. The higher the field, the better the ability to detect substances present in lower concentration and nuclei of lower sensitivity, such as ^{31}p and ^{13}C.

6.2.2 Multinuclear NMR

In addition to protons, other substances, such as ^{31}P, ^{23}Na, ^{13}C, and ^{12}F, can be detected by NMR. Electrons in orbits around the atoms modify the magnetic signal from the atom. Since hydrogen has only one orbital electron it has the greatest response to the applied magnetic field. That is, the proton experiences a greater effect than an atom with more electrons and, therefore, more atomic shielding. The electrons as they spin around the atom set up electromagnetic fields that modify the magnetic field experienced by the nucleus. Atoms are compared to protons to describe their NMR sensitivity. The sensitivity of certain atoms relative to water is given in Table 6–1.

NMR is possible because certain nuclei behave as tiny bar magnets and align themselves along magnetic lines (Figure 6–2). When a magnetic field, B_o, is applied, the spinning nuclei orient themselves either in the direction of or opposite to the applied field. If a second magnetic field is induced electronically at right angles to the originally applied field and if the new

Table 6–1. NMR Properties of Other Nuclei Compared to Hydrogen

Nucleus	Resonance Frequency at 5 T (mHz)	Spin Number	Natural Abundance (%)	Relative Sensitivity Compared to Protons
^{1}H	213.0	1/2	99.98	100
^{13}C	53.5	1/2	1.1	1.6×10^{-2}
^{15}N	21.6	1/2	0.36	3.7×10^{-4}
^{19}F	200.0	1/2	100.0	83.0
^{31}P	86.2	1/2	100.0	6.6
^{23}Na	56.3	3/2	100.0	9.3

magnetic field is oscillating at the resonant frequency, v_o, for that atom, the nuclei move up to a higher energy level.

$$\Delta E = h\,v_o \qquad\qquad (6\text{–}2)$$

where ΔE is the increase in energy and h is the Planck constant. The resonant frequency needed to excite different nuclei is determined from the magnetogyric ratio and is related to magnetic field. Each nucleus has a different magnetogyric ratio and resonates at different frequencies. The resonance frequency is related to the magnetogyric ratio by the relationship given in Equation 6–1. Since the magnetogyric ratio varies from atom to atom, for a given field there is a characteristic resonance frequency for each atom.

In a strong magnetic field, only a portion of the atoms is aligned to the field at a given time. Since millions of atoms are involved, the number actually aligned in the field direction may be only a few parts per million (ppm).

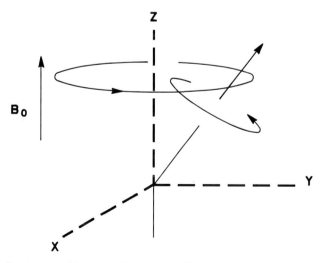

Figure 6–2. Atoms with magnetic moments line up along the magnetic field lines when placed in a magnetic field (B_0). The atoms spin about their own axis and rotate (precess) about the main axis of the field.

Homogeneous magnetic fields are needed to produce sufficient signal for spectra formation. Inhomogeneous fields degrade the signal. Inhomogeneities can be due to magnet design problems or characteristics of the sample being studied.

Each nucleus within a molecule may experience a slightly different magnetic field because the electrons within the molecule shield the nuclei from the full force of the applied field. This so-called nuclear shielding, or δ, is proportional to the applied field. In effect, the other nuclei have shifted the resonance frequency, and a new term is introduced to relate the amount of shift to a reference compound. The Larmor equation (6–1) is now written as

$$\nu_A = \gamma B_o (1 - \sigma_A)/2\pi \qquad (6\text{--}2)$$

where σ_A is the screening constant for nucleus A (Shaw, 1981). An example of the effect of nuclear shielding on the proton NMR spectrum is given in Figure 6–3. Methanol has a chemical formula of CH_3OH and contains 4 protons. In a magnetic field with homogeneity greater than 10^7, the protons near the carbon can be distinguished from those near the oxygen. The methyl protons ($-CH_3$) are shielded more than the hydroxyl protons ($-OH$). This causes the methyl protons to resonate at a lower frequency.

The chemical shift is defined as the nuclear shielding divided by the applied field. A reference compound either external to the measured material or within it is needed. The chemical shift of the nucleus A (δ_A) is given as

$$\delta_A = [(\nu_A - \nu_{ref})/\nu_{ref}] \times 10^6 \text{ ppm} \qquad (6\text{--}3)$$

here ν_{ref} is the effective frequencies experienced by a reference compound, and ν_A is that of the sample. The shielding effect produces a shift that is dimensionless and expressed in ppm. The higher the applied or reference magnetic field, the greater the separation in Hz. Two peaks with a separation of 60 Hz in a 60 mHz field (1 ppm) will be 100 Hz apart in a 100 mHz spectrometer.

Nuclear magnetism is extremely small compared to, for example, para-

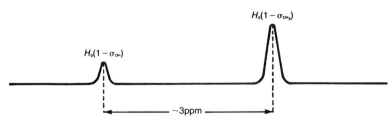

Figure 6–3. Proton NMR spectrum of methanol (CH_3OH) in a magnetic field with uniformity greater than 10^7. Two chemically shifted lines are resolved arising from the methyl and hydroxyl protons. The 3 methyl protons are 3 times higher than the 1 hydroxyl proton. (From Shaw, 1981)

magnetism, which is found in materials in which magnetic fields can be induced. Hydrogen nuclei act as tiny bar magnets in a strong magnetic field. Normally, the nuclei are aligned randomly, with some pointing up and others down. The net effect is no magnetic moment. Protons of hydrogen have spin of $1/2$ and two possible energy states. As they line up in the field, they experience a force that causes them to gyrate about their axis. The angular velocity at which they will gyrate or precess depends on the field strength and the characteristics of the nuclei. For example, hydrogen with a spin of $1/2$ has two possible positions ($2j + 1$) where j = spin number.

An NMR spectrometer works by inducing an oscillating field around the sample at a frequency that causes nuclei in the sample to resonate. When the resonating frequency induced equals the characteristic frequency for that substance, there is a transition from the lower to the higher energy state, and energy is absorbed. Normally, there is a small preponderance of nuclei that are in the lower energy state. This amounts to less than 1 part in 10^6. The slight energy absorption can be detected with a sensitive electronic amplifier. The resonance frequency causes the nuclear magnets to precess synchronously. The spectrometer detects the signals, which begin to decay with time. The original spectrometers change the magnetic field to find the resonant frequency and produce the signal. This form of NMR, called continuous NMR, was very time consuming. A major advance occurred with the use of Fourier transforms, which allow the simultaneous recording of multiple frequencies at the same magnetic field.

6.2.3 Fourier Transformation

Fourier transformation converts the signal from the time to the frequency domain (Figure 6–4). By turning the signal on and off rapidly at a time interval of t seconds, a range of frequencies centered about the original frequency, F, occurs. This is referred to as pulsed Fourier transform NMR and has become the NMR method of choice. When the pulse is applied, a single decaying curve is obtained in the time domain for each appropriate nucleus that converts to a single peak for that nucleus in the frequency domain. A pulse of time, t, produces a frequency response that has an inherent uncertainty of $1/t$. In other words, the shorter the pulse, the greater the frequency spread. Relaxation of molecules when the pulse is stopped leads to the return to the unexcited state; that is, the alignment of the nuclei in the field is lost. Relaxation to the unexcited state is referred to as T_1 relaxation. Interactions between nuclei also occur, and relaxation of the interacting nuclei is referred to as T_2 relaxation.

6.2.4 Relaxation Phenomenon and the Rotating Frame

A convenient way of thinking about relaxation phenomenon is to use the concept of the rotating frame. Earlier in the chapter, the fundamental equation (Equation 6–1) related the frequency of precession of the nuclei of a given atom to the magnetic field and the characteristic magnetogyric ratio.

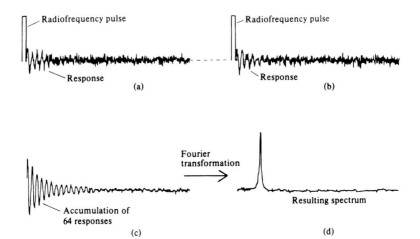

Figure 6–4. Spectrum from a single resonance are accumulated. a and b. Two consecutive responses to radiofrequency pulses of 20 msec duration and at intervals of about 1 second. c. Accumulation of 64 responses or scans. d. The spectrum obtained on Fourier transformation of the accumulation. (From Gadian, 1982)

In a magnetic field, B_o, a sample of nuclei with nuclear spin $1/2$ will precess around the direction of the field with a frequency of ν_o which is called the Larmor frequency. The nuclei will align either with or against the field (up or down). Because a slight excess of nuclei align themselves in the direction of the field, there is a resulting net magnetization in that direction, M_o. If the xy plane is set to rotate in the same direction as the precessing nuclei, they would appear stationary and could be simply described by a bulk magnetization vector. This construct is useful in imagining the effects of pulse sequences. The concepts of the rotating frame, pulse sequences, and relaxation are central to understanding biological NMR; they are discussed in greater detail by Gadian (1982).

Radiating the sample with another pulse of the same frequency as the Larmor frequency but along the y axis results in the tipping of the magnetization vector into the xy plane. When nuclei are excited by the appropriate radiofrequency pulse in a magnetic field, they have a net magnetic moment in the direction of the excitation. If we assume that the original moment is in the z direction of the xyz reference frame, relaxation back to the unexcited state takes a certain amount of time. Relaxation back to the original z plane is referred to as spin–lattice relaxation. Spin–lattice, or T_1, recovery can be measured by the inversion-recovery method (Figure 6–5). The original alignment in the field along the B_o field lines results in the alignment of the nuclei in the z direction. A pulse of radiofrequency energy of sufficient length to invert the magnetic moment $180°$ is applied. There is a waiting period of length τ, and the signal begins to recover. Another pulse of $90°$ is given, and the amount of signal that has recovered is recorded during the collection time, t_D. Signal collection occurs in the xy plane; the

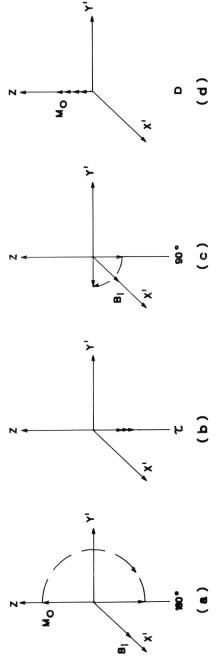

Figure 6–5. Inversion-recovery Fourier transform method for T_1 determination. a. Net magnetization in Z direction equals M_0. A 180° pulse inverts the magnetization vector. b. M_z then recovers toward its initial value M_0 during time, τ. c. A 90° pulse tilts this magnetization into the recording xy plane. The size of the resulting signal is determined by the magnetization at the time of recording. d. After a delay of time $D > 4$ T_1, the magnetization, M_z, has relaxed to its initial value of M_0, and the cycle can then be repeated.

90° pulse is needed after the 180° inversion pulse to position the signal in the correct plane. An inversion-recovery pulse sequence is given as

$$(180° - \tau - 90° - AT - D)_n$$

where AT is the acquisition time for the signal to be collected, and D is the delay between collections, which is at least 4 times the T_1 value. T_1 measurements are made by collecting spectra at different τ values and plotting the value of $\ln(M_{inf} - M_t)$ against τ. A straight line results with a slope of $1/T_1$.

The interaction between molecules is measured by the T_2 or spin–spin relaxation methods. Spin–spin measurements are more difficult to do and more subject to error than T_1. The reason for this is that inhomogeneities in the magnetic field contribute to the apparent spin–spin relaxation time. Measurement of T_2 relaxation is made by the spin–echo method (Figure 6–6). The magnetization is tilted 90° into the xy plane. The phase coherence is gradually lost because of slight inhomogeneities in the field. The inhomogeneities cause one nucleus to precess slightly faster than another nucleus in another part of the magnetic field. This results in the faster moving molecule dephasing ahead of the slower one. When the field is flipped 180°, the slower moving nuclei are placed inside the faster moving ones so that they refocus at the same time, partially correcting the effect of the inhomogeneity. After a time delay, the signal has dephased around the z axis. Another pulse of 180° reverses the dephasing signal, and continued fanning brings the signal to a focus along the y axis, forming a mirror image or echo of the original signal. The echo can be repeated a number of times at every 2t seconds. As with the T_1 measurements over time, the signal intensity at each echo is slightly less, and T_2 can be calculated from a plot of $\ln(M_y - M_y^o)$ against time.

Relaxation measurements are made after pulse sequences have been applied to help identify the origin of the signals. Bound molecules, such as those in crystals or membranes, have shorter relaxation times because they are less mobile than unbound ones. Therefore, altering the delay time before signal acquisition after the final pulse in the sequence determines the components included in the signal. For example, a long delay time removes the broad signals from bound membrane compounds, since they have relaxed early, and allows the selective acquisition of the smaller, more mobile metabolites that take longer to fully relax. This is very important in proton spectroscopy of biological systems because protons in membrane lipids overwhelm the protons from more mobile metabolites that are present in smaller amounts. Appropriate choice of delay times gives better definition of the spectra and allows more accurate peak identification.

A particular advantage of NMR is that the intensity of the NMR signal indicates the concentration of the observed nuclei. Quantities can be measured from areas under the spectral curves as determined by the integral. For example, signals from 3 protons will produce an integral 3 times as large

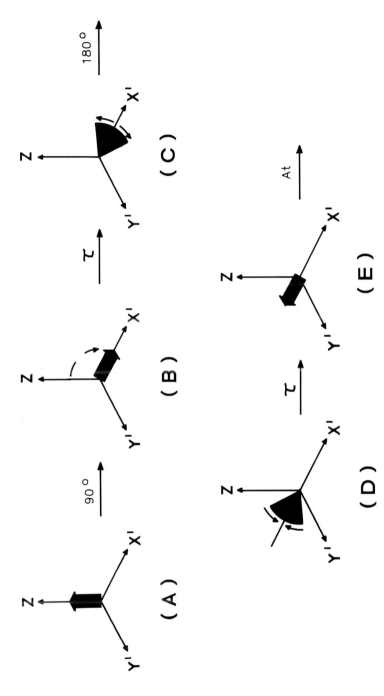

Figure 6–6. Spin–echo T_2 measurement. A. Magnetization in z direction. B. A 90° pulse tilts the magnetization onto the x'-axis. C. Field inhomogeneity causes the vector to dephase or fan out over time. D. A 180° pulse about the x'-axis reverses the magnetization. E. The precessing atoms come together or refocus into an echo during time, τ.

as from one proton. Integrals are an accurate measure of quantity, although the complexity of the spectrum often requires the use of peak heights. There are numerous problems with precise measurement of peak areas, and none of the various ways of estimating areas in chemical samples have been optimal for in vivo studies.

6.2.5 In Vivo NMR

Nuclei with greater ppm separation are more easily identified by NMR. Figure 6–7 shows the ppm spread for the three atoms of biological importance ^1H, ^{31}P, and ^{13}C. For example, the C3 carbon of lactate resonates at 21 ppm at 300 Hz, whereas the C1 carbon of glucose resonates at 96 ppm. This wide spread allows for unequivocal identification. Phosphorus-31 has a 30 ppm spread from ATP to phosphomonoesters. Protons, on the other hand, are more difficult to identify, particularly at low field strength or with inhomogeneous fields because the ppm spread is from 1 to 10, with many compounds of interest in the 1 to 4 region.

Phosphorus and proton spectroscopy have been of the greatest interest in in vivo spectroscopy because of their relatively short acquisition times. For example, ^{31}P spectra require 15–30 minutes depending on the volume sampled, whereas ^1H spectra from a rat brain at 7T can be obtained in under 10 minutes. In vivo studies have been performed with the use of surface coils (Ackerman et al., 1980), which both transmit the pulses that excite the nuclei and act as receivers for the resonating signal. The coils generally contain one or two turns. They range in size from very small coils to obtain spectra from a small portion of tissue to very large coils used to produce images in body scanners. Coil development was an important step in obtaining reliable in vivo spectra from animals.

Phosphorus spectra show the phosphorus atoms in ATP, inorganic phosphate, phosphocreatine, phosphodiesters, and phosphomonoesters. Each phosphorus atom can be identified from its chemical shift in a high-resolution ^{31}P spectrum (Figure 6–8). Studies of perchloric acid extracts have

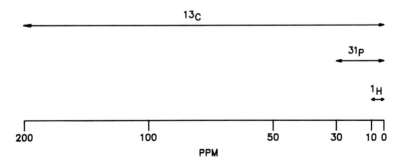

Figure 6–7. The ppm spread of ^1H, ^{31}P, and ^{13}C is shown. ^{13}C has the greatest spread and the more readily resolved spectrum, whereas ^1H with the smallest spread is most difficult to resolve.

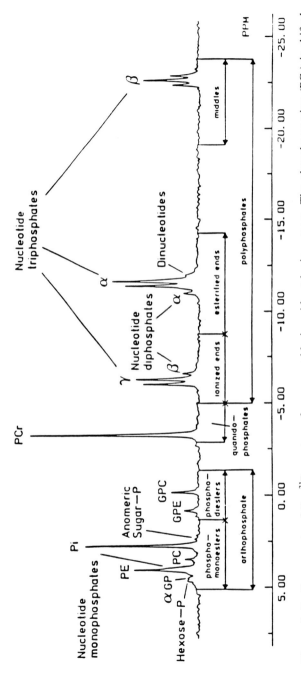

Figure 6–8. Components of the ^{31}P spectrum from a perchloric acid rat brain extract. The phosphocreatine (PCr) is shifted from the usual internal reference at 0.00 ppm. The abbreviations are given in Table 6–2. (From Pettegrew et al., 1989)

shown the ^{31}P components in the NMR spectra (Glonek et al., 1982; Gyulai et al., 1984). Phosphocreatinine (PCr) is used as the ppm reference standard at 0.00 ppm. The phosphomonoester region is from 5 to 1.5 ppm, and the phosphodiester region from 1.5 to -1.5 ppm. The polyphosphate region contains the γ-, α-, and β-ATP phosphates along with the nucleotide diphosphate. The β-ATP is the only ATP resonance that has no contribution from the dinucleotides.

Phosphoesters are shown in Table 6–2. The phosphomonoesters contain the major brain phospholipids: phosphatidylethanolamine, phosphatidylcholine, and α-glycerylphosphate. These are found mainly in anabolic pathways, whereas the phosphodiesters GPE and GPC are important in catabolic pathways. The ratio of phosphomonesters to phosphodiesters has been proposed as an approximation of brain phospholipid turnover (Pettegrew et al., 1988).

In vivo proton NMR has been obtained only recently because of the need to suppress the large proton signal from water. Pulse sequences have been designed that suppress the overwhelming water signal and reveal protons on other molecules of biological interest found in lower concentrations. Water suppression is possible because of differential relaxation properties among various protons. By proper selection of the pulse sequences, the large water signal, or any solvent signal, can be suppressed and the signal of interest moved into the recording plane. For example, protons on water relax in the z axis after a 180° pulse, moving toward the zero point in the xy plane. Another, more slowing relaxing substance will be below the xy plane when the water is at zero, and its signal is nullified. If a second 90° pulse is applied when the water is in the zero position, the molecule of interest will be tilted into the xy plane, and its relaxation will be recorded. Thus, a (180°–τ–90°) pulse sequence can be used to suppress water (Figure 6–9).

The relaxation behavior of large molecules is complex. This becomes important in identifying signals from lipids. Fatty acids have a large number of protons. Under normal conditions, the majority of fatty acids are relatively immobile within the lipid backbone of the membrane. Within the phospholipid structure, however, the protons farther away from the binding site will be more mobile. Thus, the relaxation characteristics for different protons bonds will be different. Saturation affects the mobility and packing of the membrane, so that unsaturated fatty acids will appear more mobile. Theoretically, a change in membrane fluidity will produce an increased signal from the protons on the more mobile fatty acids. These dynamic changes may or may not reflect an actual biochemical change.

Proton NMR has been useful in the analysis of effects on membranes (Hitzemann et al., 1986). Membranes are composed of large triglyceride molecules with fatty acid side chains. The rate of relaxation of the protons in different parts of the complex lipid molecule depends on the amount of motion in the side chain. Substances, such as ethanol, which increase membrane fluidity, increase ^{1}H-NMR relaxation times for lipids. In other words,

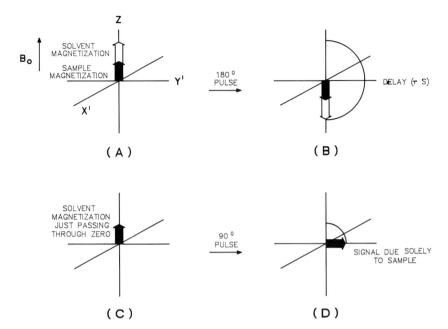

Figure 6–9. Solvent suppression pulse sequence. A. The solvent and sample are magnetized. B. A 180° pulse tilts them both into the negative z plane. C. After a delay of seconds, the solvent magnetization passes through zero. D. The sample is tilted 90° into the y plane for recording of the spectrum. (From Abraham and Loftus, 1978)

the greater the ability of the proton to move within the membrane, the more prolonged the relaxation time.

The mobility of long chains has been well studied with ^{13}C-NMR. For example, in the decane molecule, the T_1 values at each carbon bond will be determined by the mobility at that specific bond (Abraham and Loftus, 1978). The greatest mobility is at the ends, with reduced movement toward the center. The decane molecule with T_1 values for ^{13}C listed above the bonds is

$$\begin{array}{ccccc} 8.7 & 6.6 & 5.7 & 5.0 & 4.4 \\ CH_3 - & CH_2 - & CH_2 - & CH_2 - & CH_2 - & C_5H_{11} \end{array}$$

where the higher numbers represent greater mobility. For a phospholipid in membranes, the ^{13}C T_1 values are important in determining the segmental motion that is related to molecular transport. If the fatty acid chain is shortened or a double bond is introduced, there is an increase in the segmental motion within the chain. The effect of shortening a fatty acid chain or introducing a double bond is shown in Figure 6–10. Membrane fluidity in-

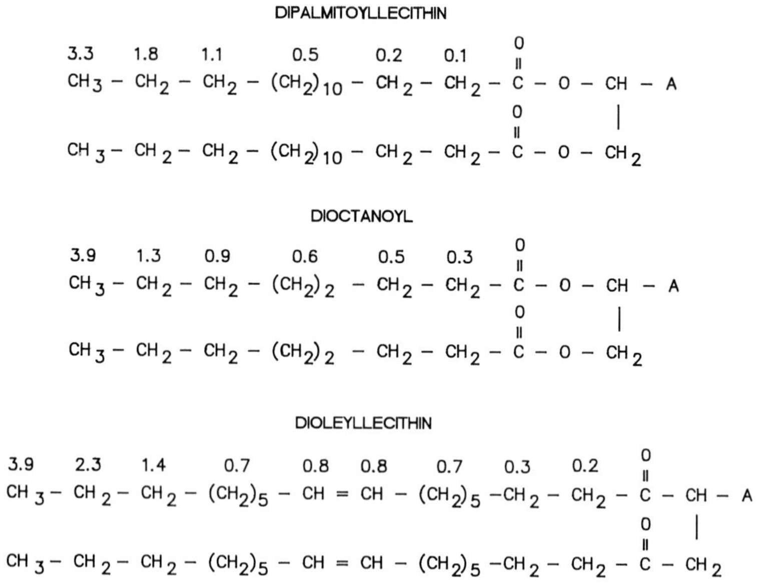

DIPALMITOYLLECITHIN

3.3   1.8   1.1   0.5   0.2   0.1   O
$CH_3 - CH_2 - CH_2 - (CH_2)_{10} - CH_2 - CH_2 - \overset{\overset{O}{\|}}{C} - O - CH - A$

$CH_3 - CH_2 - CH_2 - (CH_2)_{10} - CH_2 - CH_2 - \overset{\overset{O}{\|}}{C} - O - CH_2$

DIOCTANOYL

3.9   1.3   0.9   0.6   0.5   0.3
$CH_3 - CH_2 - CH_2 - (CH_2)_2 - CH_2 - CH_2 - \overset{\overset{O}{\|}}{C} - O - CH - A$

$CH_3 - CH_2 - CH_2 - (CH_2)_2 - CH_2 - CH_2 - \overset{\overset{O}{\|}}{C} - O - CH_2$

DIOLEYLLECITHIN

3.9   2.3   1.4   0.7   0.8   0.8   0.7   0.3   0.2
$CH_3 - CH_2 - CH_2 - (CH_2)_5 - CH = CH - (CH_2)_5 - CH_2 - CH_2 - \overset{\overset{O}{\|}}{C} - CH - A$

$CH_3 - CH_2 - CH_2 - (CH_2)_5 - CH = CH - (CH_2)_5 - CH_2 - CH_2 - \overset{\overset{O}{\|}}{C} - CH_2$

Figure 6–10. The effect of shortening a fatty acid chain or introducing a double bond is shown for phospholipids: Dipalmitoyllecithin, dioctanoyl, dioleyllecithin. The effect of increasing segmental motion at the end of the chemicals is shown. The numbers represent T_1 measurements; the higher numbers indicate greater mobility. (From Abraham and Loftus, 1978)

creases as the segmental motion along the chain increases. Thus, it is possible to follow in vivo changes in membrane fluidity with NMR.

6.3 ^{31}P-NMR

6.3.1 In Vitro ^{31}P-NMR

Of the nuclei used for in vivo spectroscopy, ^{1}H, ^{19}F, and ^{31}P are 100 percent abundant, whereas ^{13}C is only 1.1 percent. Because of its natural abundance, ubiquitous presence in all biological tissue, and favorable ppm spread, ^{31}P-NMR was the first to be applied successfully to whole organisms in vivo (Ackerman et al., 1980).

Phosphorus can be used to follow high-energy phosphate metabolism and to measure pH shifts. PCr is used as the standard to measure the chemical shifts of inorganic phosphate and to calculate pH. As the pH falls, the chemical shift difference between inorganic phosphate and PCr narrows (Figure 6–11). Measurement of pH with ^{31}P-NMR has been an important application of in vivo NMR. The chemical shift difference between P_i and PCr is affected by pH and various paramagnetic substances, such as magnesium. The equation for calculating brain pH at magnesium concentrations of 2.5 mM or less is (Petroff et al., 1985)

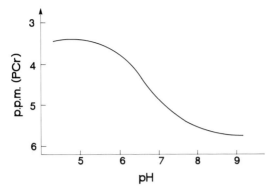

Figure 6–11. The ppm or chemical shift difference between inorganic phosphate and phosphocreatinine (PCr) plotted against pH. 10 mM PCr titrated at 37°C by addition for HCl and KOH. (From Gadian, 1982)

$$pH = 6.77 + \log[(\delta - 3.29)/(5.68 - \delta)] \qquad (6\text{–}4)$$

Initial studies of ^{31}P metabolism with NMR were done in muscle because limbs could be fit into the small bore of available magnets and had high levels of phosphorus-containing compounds (Hoult et al., 1974). To obtain these signals in living organisms, surface coils have been designed to provide both the exciting electromagnetic field and to act as the recording antenna. Surface coils focus on a small volumn below the coils with special pulse sequences.

The conversion of ATP to ADP and inorganic phosphate (P_i) is the main source of energy for biosynthesis, osmotic work, and active transport in the cell.

$$ATP + H_2O = ADP + P_i + H^+$$
$$G° = -7,000 \ cal/mol \qquad (6\text{–}5)$$

The energy released is large and normally coupled to cellular work rather than released as heat. ATP can transfer a phosphate group to creatine (Cr), which can be stored in cells in the form of PCr,

$$ATP + Cr + H^+ = ADP + PCr \qquad (6\text{–}6)$$

Thus, PCr can be accessed rapidly in tissue, such as muscle, where it serves as a high-energy buffer to maintain ATP levels during exercise. Glycolysis and oxidative phosphorylation provide the long-term energy source for cells in either anaerobic or aerobic conditions.

$$Glycogen + P_i + ADP = ATP + lactic \ acid \qquad (6\text{–}7)$$
$$Glycogen/glucose + ADP + P_i + O_2 = ATP + H_2O + CO_2 \quad (6\text{–}8)$$

The chemical shifts and concentrations of these various sources of energy can be measured with ^{31}P-NMR.

6.3.2 In Vivo ^{31}P-NMR

Initial studies of in vivo metabolism performed with ^{31}P-NMR in muscle provided an opportunity to confirm biochemical studies of phosphorus metabolism. The equilibrium of ATP formation from PCr by creatine kinase implies that ADP would be found at a very low level. This was indeed observed in studies of muscle, thus confirming the biochemical results (Veech et al., 1979).

An initial study demonstrating the usefulness of NMR spectroscopy was done in a patient with a rare muscle disease, McArdle's syndrome (Ross et al., 1981). These patients have a deficiency of the enzyme phosphorylase, which catalyzes the breakdown of glycogen. This enzyme defect leads to exercise intolerance in the patient. Normal subjects maintain PCr and ATP levels during ischemic exercise, whereas patients with McArdle's syndrome show a dramatic loss of PCr and gain of P_i during ischemic exercise. Furthermore, the generation of lactic acid under anaerobic conditions in normal subjects results in a fall in intracellular pH, whereas the lack of lactic acid production in patients with McArdle's syndrome prevented the normal drop in the pH of muscle.

Another example of NMR spectroscopy in diagnosing muscle disease was reported in a child with a mitochondrial myopathy. The patient had, in addition, an ophthalmoplegia and raised basal metabolic rate. At rest, he had a mild lactic acidosis with blood lactate of 3 mmol/liter, which reached a peak of 17 mmol/liter with sustained exercise. At rest, the NMR muscle spectrum showed a reduction of the normal PCr/P_i ratio, with a normal intracellular pH. As opposed to the McArdle's syndrome patient, the response to aerobic exercise with a fall in blood pH was normal. The high concentration of P_i at rest may be considered a direct consequence of the lesion in oxidative phosphorylation (Gadian, 1982).

^{31}P-NMR is used to study in vivo brain metabolism (Thulborn et al., 1982; Cady et al., 1983; Petroff et al., 1985; Bottomley et al., 1986; Welch et al., 1989). The normal spectrum from brain shows peaks from ATP, PCr, phosphomonesters and phosphodiesters, and inorganic phosphate (Figure 6–12).

Table 6–2. Molecules Contributing to the Phosphoester Region in Brain ^{31}P-NMR Spectra

Phosphomonester Region	Phosphodiester Region
Hexose-6-phosphate (hexose-P)	Glycerol 3-phosphoethanolamine (GPE)
Phosphoethanolamine (PE)	Glycerol 3-phosphocholine (GPC)
Phosphocholine (PC)	Phosphorylated glycolipids
α-Glycerylphosphate (α-GP)	Glycoproteins
Inorganic phosphate (P_i)	

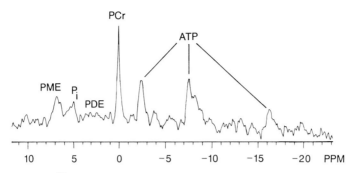

Figure 6–12. A ^{31}P-NMR spectrum obtained from a volume of rat brain with a surface coil in a 7 Tesla 89 mm bore spectrometer. Peaks are phosphomonoesters (PME), inorganic phosphate (P$_i$), phosphodiesters (PDE), phosphocreatinine, (PCr), and adenosine triphosphate (ATP).

6.4 ^{13}C-NMR

The ^{13}C molecule has a spin of $1/2$ and a natural abundance of 1.1 percent. Compared to protons, its sensitivity is 1.6×10^{-2} at natural abundance concentrations. Spectra have been obtained from natural abundance measurements, but in most circumstances, it is necessary to enrich the ^{13}C for detection in biological tissue within a reasonable time (Prichard and Shulman, 1986). Enrichment is possible by synthesizing compounds labeled with ^{13}C. By injecting labeled substances in animals, it is possible to follow metabolic processes without extensive biochemical analyses.

The wide ppm range for ^{13}C provides a method to identify the position of the ^{13}C atom in a molecule. This is helpful in natural abundance studies where chemical structure can be determined. More important for biological studies, however, is the ability to use enriched molecules as tracers. In this respect, the low natural abundance of ^{13}C is an asset. A ^{13}C spectrum from glutamate and GABA is shown in Figure 6–13. Each atom has a unique ppm signal so that full identification is possible.

Injection of glucose with a ^{13}C molecule in the 1 position, 1-^{13}C-glucose, into animals results in incorporation of the ^{13}C into brain glycolytic and nonglycolytic metabolites. The ^{13}C labeled in the 1 position appears in the lactate labeled in the C3 position (Figure 6–14). After entering the Krebs cycle, it is incorporated into the C4 position of glutamate, and with subsequent turns it is seen also in the C2 and C3 positions.

Following the injection of 1-^{13}C-glucose intravenously into rat, the tracer is seen in several compounds after 30 minutes (Figure 6–15). Although long collection times are necessary for ^{13}C analysis of a single rat brain, it is possible to shorten considerably the collection time by combining several brains for analysis. These studies are usually done in chemically extracted brain tissue because of the difficulty of detecting ^{13}C-labeled metabolites in vivo. The ^{13}C molecule normally is present in 1.1 percent of carbon atoms.

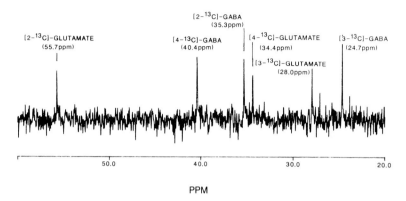

Figure 6–13. A ^{13}C-NMR spectrum from γ-Aminobutyric acid (GABA) and glutamate. The various atoms within the molecule are identified, and the ppm chemical shift is labeled. Compounds were run in solution on a Brucker WM-300 NMR spectrometer. Samples were dissolved in 20 percent D_2O and adjusted to pH 7.4. Spectra accumulated using a 45° tip angle, 1.16 second pulse interval. Chemical shifts are given relative to tetramethylsilane (TMS). (Courtesy of Dr. J. Brainard, Los Alamos National Laboratory)

Enrichment with ^{13}C-labeled compounds enhances the signal, but the cost of ^{13}C compounds is high, making these studies expensive.

The sensitivity of ^{13}C detection is enhanced by the use of heteronuclear decoupling. The protons coupled to ^{13}C molecules produce a signal that differs from protons coupled to ^{12}C. The method enables the measurement of ^{1}H after irradiation of ^{13}C. If the protons on ^{13}C are decoupled, they can be detected with those on ^{12}C, and by subtracting the results of the coupled and decoupled spectra, the protons on ^{13}C can be determined. The ^{1}H observe–^{13}C decouple method has been used to follow glutamate labeling with ^{13}C in rat brain (Rothman et al., 1985). Techniques such as these, along with improvements in ^{13}C surface coils, may make ^{13}C measurements in humans possible.

6.5 ^{1}H-NMR

6.5.1 In Vitro ^{1}H-NMR

A ^{1}H-NMR spectrum contains numerous compounds of importance in metabolism studies. At high field strengths, separation of these compounds by ^{1}H-NMR is possible. A ^{1}H-NMR spectrum of a perchloric acid extract from an animal whose brain was rapidly frozen with liquid nitrogen in situ under normal oxygen conditions is shown in Figure 6–16. The methyl group of lactate resonates at 1.33 ppm. The major proton signal comes from the abun-

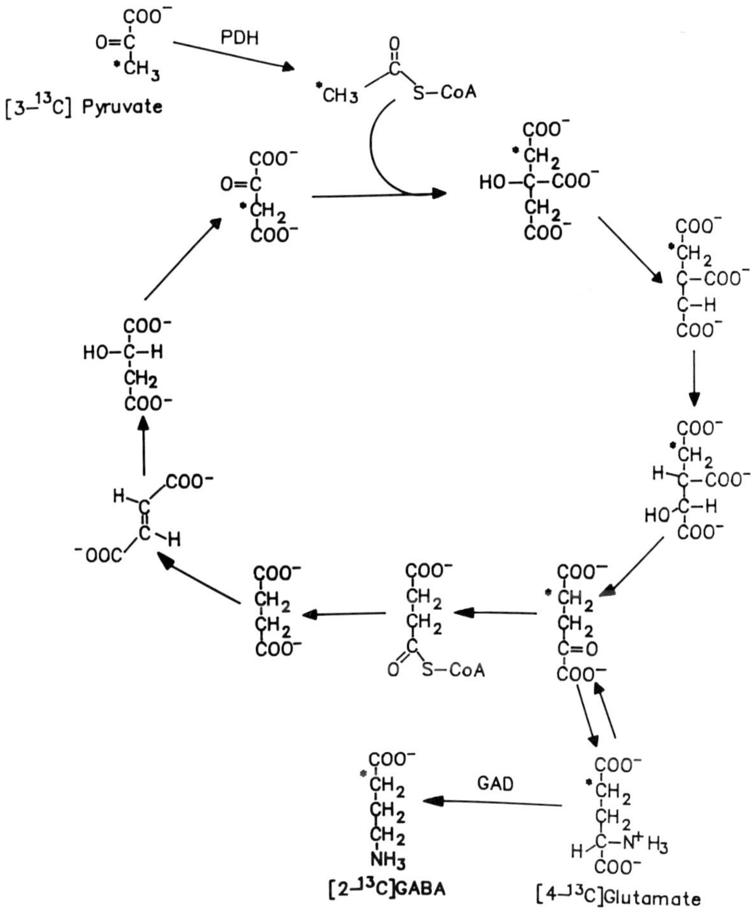

Figure 6–14. The metabolism of 1-^{13}C-glucose in the tricarboxylic acid cycle is shown. The label (*) initially in the C1 position of glucose is metabolized by pyruvate dehydrogenase (PDH) into the C4 position of glutamate and the C2 position of GABA.

dant water in brain. Protons from other compounds are obscured by the large water signal. However, pulse sequences have been developed that suppress the water protons (Hore, 1983). Metabolites present in millimolar concentrations can be detected in vivo in brain by proton NMR with water suppression. Table 6–3 gives the ppm for some ^{1}H-NMR metabolites found in brain.

The perchloric acid extraction procedure removes the lipids and preserves carbohydrates and amino acids. The peaks have been identified by the presence of characteristic bonds (Arus et al., 1985; Fan et al., 1986). Identification of molecules is possible by NMR, although several protons can have similar bonds, and there may be overlapping of the resonance peaks in the spectrum obtained. For example, protons attached to different carbon atoms in the glutamate molecule produce peaks at 2.0 and 2.3 ppm. N-Acetyl groups

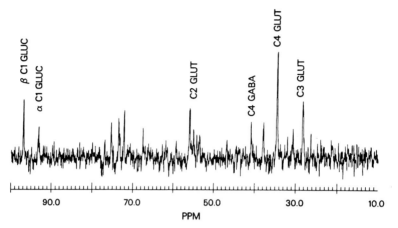

Figure 6–15. ^{13}C NMR spectrum of brain extract obtained 30 minutes after 1-^{13}C-glucose injection. The major metabolic products are C4 glutamate (glut) from one turn through the TCA cycle and C2 glut and C3 glut from a second turn. Two forms of glucose (gluc) are seen. Analyzed as described in Figure 6–13. (Courtesy of Dr. J. Brainard, Los Alamos National Laboratory)

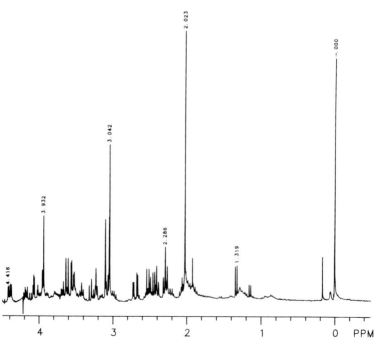

Figure 6–16. ^{1}H-NMR spectrum from a perchloric acid extract of a normal rat brain. The sample was dissolved in D$_2$O after freeze-drying and analyzed at 7 T. The bonds forming the various peaks are given in Table 6–3.

114

Table 6–3. Characteristic ^{1}H-NMR Peaks in a Spectrum from a Perchloric Acid Brain Extract

Compound	Bond	ppm	Splitting[a]
β-Hydroxybutyrate	β-CH$_3$	1.23	d
Lactate	β-CH$_3$	1.34	d
Alanine	β-CH$_3$	1.47	d
GABA	β-CH$_2$	1.88	m
Acetate	CH$_3$	1.91	s
NAA	NA$_c$CH$_3$	2.02	s
Glutamate	β-CH$_2$	2.14	c
GABA	α-CH$_2$	2.23	t
Glutamate	γ-CH$_2$	2.34	t
Succinate	—(CH$_2$)—$_2$	2.40	s
Glutamate	γ-CH$_2$	2.45	c
NAA	β-CH$_2$	2.65	d
GABA	γ-CH$_2$	3.00	t
PCR/CR	CH$_3$	3.07	s
PCR/CR	CH$_2$	3.92	s
Lactate	α-CH	4.12	q

[a]d, doublet; m, multiplet; s, singlet; c, complex; t, triplet; q, quadruplet. NAA = N-Acetylaspartate.
(From Fan et al., 1986).

resonate at 2.0 ppm. The methyl protons on lactate have a unique resonance at 1.3 ppm. Concentrations of these substances can reach millimolar amounts so that in vivo detection is theoretically possible.

Lipids form a high percentage of brain tissue. The membrane-bound lipids produce a broad signal in vivo in the region of the lactate signal. Since this is undesirable for some studies of brain lactate, pulse sequences are used that either have longer delay times to allow the bound lipid molecules to relax, or have a delay time set to invert the lactate signal. Bound lipids remain undetected, whereas signals from more mobile lipids may still be present at longer delay times. These lipids have been poorly characterized but may represent those that are part of the membrane cytoskeleton or suspended in the cytosol or extracellular space.

6.5.2 In Vivo ^{1}H-NMR

One method of studying brain metabolism involves obtaining spectra from regions below the skull by the use of depth selective pulse sequences. These are pulse sequences that focus on a region below the surface (Bendall and Gordon, 1983).

Combining the depth pulse sequences with water suppression provides a means to follow in vivo brain metabolism. At low field strength, such as 2T, studies in animals have been used to analyze lactate changes (Behar et al. 1984). There is a large lipid signal in the region of lactate that can be removed by spectral editing methods (Williams et al., 1988) or by use of long spin–echo delay times that allow the less mobile membrane lipids to decay away. Selective lactate editing has been used to study brain pH and

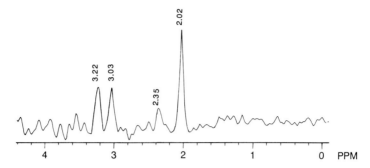

Figure 6–17. In-vivo ¹H-NMR spectra from an anesthetized rat in a 7 Tesla GN300 spectrometer with an 89-mm bore. The spectra is obtained with a Bendall depth pulse using water supression. The spin-echo delay was 280 msec. Peaks are numbered and shown in Table 6–3.

lactate simultaneously. An in vivo spectrum from an anesthetized rat in a 7 T 89 mm bore magnet is shown in Figure 6–17. The spectrum during life corresponds to the spectrum from a perchloric acid extract (Figure 6–16).

The in vivo ¹H-NMR spectrum obtained with surface coils and water suppression in animals contains information about brain amino acids, lipids, and lactate. The manner in which the spectra are collected determines the type of information obtained. Optimal spectra are obtained with spin–echo pulse sequences. The longer the spin–echo delay time, the more mobile the metabolites observed.

REFERENCES

Abraham, R. J., Loftus, P.: *Proton and Carbon-13 NMR Spectroscopy: An Integrated Approach*. Chichester, England: John Wiley & Sons, 1978.

Ackerman, J. J. H., Grove, T. H., Wong, G. G., Gadian, D. G., Radda G. K.: Mapping of metabolites in whole animals by ³¹P-NMR using surface coils. Nature 283:167–170, 1980.

Arus, C., Yen-Chang, Barany, M.: Proton nuclear magnetic resonance spectra of excised rat brain. Assignment of resonances. Physiol. Chem. Physics Med. NMR 17:23–33, 1985.

Behar, K. L., Rothman, D. L., Shulman, R. G., Petroff, O. A., Prichard, J. W.: Detection of cerebral lactate in vivo during hypoxemia by ¹H-NMR at relatively low field strengths (1.9 T). Proc. Natl. Acad. Sci. USA 81:2517–2519, 1984.

Bendall, M. R., Gordon, R. E.: Depth and refocusing pulses designed for multipulse NMR with surface coils. J. Magn. Reson. 53:365–385, 1983.

Bottomley, P. A., Drayer, B. P., Smith, L. S.: Chronic adult cerebral infarction studied by phosphorus NMR spectroscopy. Radiology 160:763–766, 1986.

Budinger, T. F., Lauterbur, P. C.: Nuclear magnetic resonance technology for medical studies. Science 226:288–298, 1984.

Cady, E. B., Costello, A. M., Dawson, M. J., Delpy, D. T., Hope, P. L., Reynolds, E. O., Tofts, P. S., Wilkie, D. R.: Non-invasive investigation of cerebral metabolism in newborn infants by phosphorus nuclear magnetic resonance spectroscopy. Lancet 1:1059–1062, 1983.

Fan, T. W. M., Higashi, R. M., Lane, A. N., Jardetsky, O.: Combined use of ^{1}H-NMR and GC-MS for metabolite monitoring and in vivo ^{1}H-NMR assignments. Biochim. Biophys. Acta. 882:154–167, 1986.

Gadian, D. G.: *Nuclear Magnetic Resonance and Its Application to Living Systems.* Oxford: Oxford University Press, 1982.

Glonek, T., Kopp, S., Kot, E., Pettegrew, J., Harrison, W., Cohen, M.: ^{31}P-Nuclear resonance analysis of brain. I. The perchloric acid extract spectrum. J. Neurochem. 39:1210–1219, 1982.

Gyulai, L., Bolinger, L., Leigh, J. S., Jr, Barlow, C., Chance, B.: Phosphorylethanolamine—The major constituent of the phosphomonoester peak observed by ^{31}P-NMR on developing dog brain. FEBS Lett. 178:137–142, 1984.

Hitzemann, R. J., Schueler, H. E., Graham-Brittain, C., Kreishman, G. P.: Ethanol-induced changes in neuronal membrane order. An NMR study. Biochim. Biophys. Acta. 859:189–197, 1986.

Hore, P. J.: Solvent supression in fourier transform nuclear magnetic resonance. J. Magn. Reson. 55:283–300, 1983.

Hoult, D. I., Busby, S. J. W., Gadian, D. G., Radda, G. K., Richards, R. E., Seeley, P. J.: Observation of tissue metabolites using ^{31}P nuclear magnetic resonance. Nature 252:285–287, 1974.

Lauterbur, P. C.: Image formation by induced local interactions: Examples employing nuclear magnetic resonance. Nature 242:190–191, 1973.

Petroff, O. A., Prichard, J. W., Behar, K. L., Alger, J. R., den Hollander, J. A., Shulman, R. G.: Cerebral intracellular pH by ^{31}P nuclear magnetic resonance spectroscopy. Neurology 35:781–788, 1985.

Pettegrew, J. W., Moossy, J., Withers, G., McKeag, D., Panchalingam, K.: [31]P nuclear magnetic resonance study of the brain in Alzheimer's disease. J. Neuropathol. Exp. Neurol. 47:235–248, 1988.

Pettegrew, J. W., Withers, G., Panchalingam, K.: ^{31}P-NMR of brain aging and Alzheimers disease. In *Nuclear Magnetic Resonance: The Principles and Applications of NMR Spectroscopy and Imaging to Biomedical Research.* Pettegrew, J. W., ed. New York: Springer-Verlag, 1990:204–254.

Prichard, J. W., Shulman, R. G.: NMR spectroscopy of brain metabolism in vivo. Annu. Rev. Neurosci. 9:61–85, 1986.

Ross, B. D., Radda, G. K., Gadian, D. G., Rocker, G., Esiri, M., Falconer Smith, J.: Examination of a case of suspected McArdle's syndrome by ^{31}P nuclear magnetic resonance. N. Engl. J. Med. 304:1338–1342, 1981.

Rothman, D. L., Behar, K. L., Hetherington, H. P., den Hollander, J. A., Bendall, M. R., Petroff, O. A., Shulman, R. G.: [1]H-observe/^{13}C-decouple spectroscopic measurements of lactate and glutamate in the rat brain in vivo. Proc. Natl. Acad. Sci. USA 82:1633–1637, 1985.

Shaw, D.: In *Nuclear Magnetic Resonance Imaging in Medicine.* Kaufman, L., Crooks, L. E., Margulis, A. R., eds. New York: Igaku-Shoin, 1981:147.

Thulborn, D. R., duBoulay, G. H., Duchen, L. W., Radda, G. K.: A ^{31}P nuclear magnetic resonance in vivo study of cerebral ischaemia in the gerbil. J. Cerebr. Blood Flow Metab. 2:299–306, 1982.

Veech, R. L., Lawson, J. W., Cornell, N. W., Krebs, H. A.: Cytosolic phosphorylation potential. J. Biol. Chem. 254:6538–6547, 1979.

Welch, K. M., Levine, S. R., DAndrea, G., Schulta, L. R., Helpern, J. A.: Preliminary observations on brain energy metabolism in migraine studied by in vivo phosphorus 31 NMR spectroscopy. Neurology 39:538–541, 1989.

Williams, S. R., Proctor, E., Allen, K., Gadian, D. G., Crockard, H. A.: Quantitative estimation of lactate in the brain of ^{1}H NMR. Magn. Reson. Med. 7:425–431, 1988.

7

Glucose, Amino Acids, and Lipids

7.1 BLOOD-BRAIN BARRIER

Computed tomography, MRI, and PET have made analysis of blood–brain barrier function and glucose metabolism clinically available. Contrast agents are able to show lesions in barrier function with CT and MRI. Positron emission tomography has been able to show both transport into the brain from the blood of compounds, such as rubidium, and metabolism of glucose. Using PET scanning, new information has been obtained on the pathophysiology of various disease states. Magnetic resonance spectroscopy has shown dynamic in vivo changes in brain metabolism. Interpretation of the results of these studies requires an understanding of the central role of the blood–brain barrier in regulating the brain microenvironment and of the metabolism of glucose, amino acids, and lipids by the brain.

The blood–brain barrier is composed of a series of interfaces that separate brain tissue from the general circulation (see Chapter 2). The characteristic feature of each interface is the tight junctions that join together the epithelial cells. Cerebral capillaries form the most important interface because of their extensive surface area when compared to the other interfaces. Endothelial cells are separated from the astrocytic end-feet by the basal lamina. The astrocyte–basal lamina–endothelial cell complex functions as a unit to preserve the ionic composition of the fluid surrounding the neurons. Multiple transport systems and enzymes act in concert with the tight junctions to control the entrance of substances into the brain (Rapoport, 1976; Bradbury, 1979). Those substances that can dissolve in the membrane can cross from the blood into the brain, and, therefore, lipid-soluble substances cross the endothelial cells more readily than do ions and polar molecules, which are restricted by the tight junctions. Electron microscopic studies with the electron-dense protein, horseradish peroxidase (HRP), have shown that HRP is

prevented from leaving the blood vessel by the tight junctions between endothelial cells (Reese and Karnovsky, 1969). In the choroid plexus, there
are fenestrated capillaries that resemble those found systemically, and the
tight junctions are found instead at the apical surface of the epithelial cells.
Except for some substances, such as sodium, which more readily crosses
the choroid plexus epithelium than the capillary and selectively accumulates
in periventricular regions, the capillary transport systems are the main factor
in fluid balance.

The effectiveness of an epithelial membrane in preventing the passage of
certain substances is best determined by its electrical resistance. The tighter
the junctions, the higher the resistance they can maintain. Measurements of
the cerebral capillary electrical resistance have recorded values of 1,900 ohm/
cm^2 for frog cerebral vessels, which are in the same range as frog skin
(Crone and Christensen, 1981; Crone and Olesen, 1982). For comparison,
the very tight-junctioned urinary bladder epithelium has a resistance of 3,800
ohm/cm^2, indicating that brain capillaries behave as tight junctions and would
be impermeable to small ions. The electrical resistance of a muscle capillary
is 20 ohm/cm^2, and that of the mesenteric capillary is 1–2 ohm/cm^2. In
addition to the tight junctions, brain capillaries contain enzymes that effectively metabolize various substrates before they are allowed to enter the brain.
These enzymes include alkaline phosphatase, pseudocholinesterase, aromatic L-amino acid decarboxylase, and gamma-glutamyl transpeptidase
(Bradbury, 1984).

Understanding the mechanisms of transport of substances from blood to
brain is of great clinical importance. It has influenced concepts of disease
pathogenesis and helped in drug design. Brain capillaries have unique features that are shown schematically in Figure 7–1. The capillary is a meta-
bolically active cell involved in diverse transport functions. The high content
of mitochondria provides the energy for the transport of glucose, amino acids,
and other substances as well as the energy for the function of the Na^+,K^+-
ATPase on the abluminal surface. Astrocytic end-feet that abut on the capillary are important in fluid balance, since they swell under certain pathological conditions, such as hypoxia. The basal lamina may provide structural
support for the endothelial cell and act as a charge barrier as in other organs.
Thus, the cerebral capillary is central to normal brain function (Bradbury
and Stulcova, 1970; Goldstein and Betz, 1983).

Several factors control the transport of substances across the blood–brain
barrier, including molecular weight, extent of ionization, lipid solubility,
and carrier mechanisms. Lipid-soluble molecules pass more easily through
the endothelial cell than do nonlipid compounds. This may be either through
lipoprotein pores in the membrane or by dissolving in the membrane matrix.
For example, gases, such as oxygen, carbon dioxide, and anesthetic agents,
are highly lipid soluble and readily cross the membrane, whereas slow passage across the blood–brain barrier of certain drugs limits their therapeutic
usefulness. Modifying molecules to increase their lipid solubility has been
used to design drugs of greater therapeutic effectiveness. The octanol/water

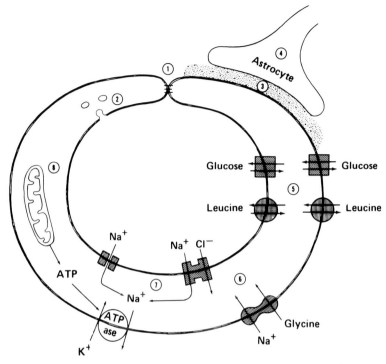

Figure 7–1. Model of brain capillary. The tight junctions (1) that join endothelial cells together in brain capillaries are continuous and complex, and they limit the diffusion of large and small solutes. Very few pinocytotic vesicles (2) are found in the cytoplasm, and this potential route for transendothelial transport is not operative in normal brain capillaries. The basement membrane (3) provides structural support for the capillary and may influence endothelial cell function. Foot processes of astrocytes (4) encircle the capillary but do not create a permeability barrier. Transport carriers (5) for glucose and essential amino acids facilitate the movement of these solutes into brain. Active transport systems (6) appear to cause efflux of certain small amino acids from brain to blood. Na^+ pores and NaCl carriers on the luminal surface of the endothelial cell and Na^+, K^+-ATPase on the antiluminal surface account for ion movements across the brain capillary (7). Mitochondria (8) produce the ATP needed for energy-dependent transport processes. Not shown are receptor sites for agents that may regulate the permeability of this barrier. (From Goldstein and Betz, 1983)

ratio of a substance is a good index of the ease of movement across the blood–brain barrier (Figure 7–2). Lipid-soluble compounds partition into the octanol, whereas nonlipids are dissolved mainly in the water. Aminopyrine is highly lipid soluble and has a partition coefficient greater than 1, whereas sucrose is very insoluble in octanol and has a very low coefficient. Modification of morphine to heroin increases its lipid solubility and enhances its entrance into the brain from the blood. Substances with low permeability remain in the blood; they provide markers of the vascular space.

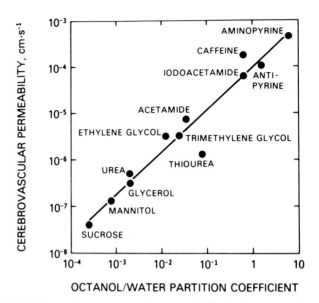

Figure 7–2. Relation of cerebrovascular permeability in the parietal cortex to octanol/water partition coefficient for 12 nonelectrolytes. Each point represents a mean for 3–5 rats. The line is the least-squares fit to the data. (From Takasato et al., 1984)

Very permeable compounds cross immediately into the brain to indicate the rate of blood flow. There are important therapeutic implications of the oil/water partition coefficients.

Treatment with penicillin is an example of the role of the blood–brain barrier in therapy. The antibiotic enters brain slowly, and very large doses are needed to reach therapeutic levels in brain tissue. However, ampicillin, chloramphenicol, and the new generation of cephalosporins penetrate into brain more readily than does penicillin and are useful in the treatment of brain infections. Occasionally, an infection with a bacterium or fungus is sensitive only to a poorly permeable antibiotic. In the treatment of coccidioidomycosis with amphotericin, it is necessary to bypass the blood–brain barrier by direct injection of the antibiotic into the CSF of the lumbar sac or intraventricularly with a ventricular cannula. Chemotherapy for brain tumors is another example of interference of the blood–brain barrier in treatment. The anticancer drug, methotrexate, is used to treat brain tumors and childhood leukemia. However, it crosses the blood–brain barrier slowly, so that either high systemic doses or intrathecal injection is needed.

Transplantation studies have shown that the stimulus for a capillary to form a tight junction comes from the brain. This was shown in transplantation studies using quail brains that have specific markers for capillaries so they can be identified and distinguished from other capillaries. Transplantation studies in which systemic capillaries are placed in quail brain show that capillaries with tight junctions are induced, presumably by the astrocytes present in brain tissue (Stewart and Wiley, 1981).

Another unique aspect of the cerebral capillary is the high content of a number of enzymes and receptors (Table 7–1). These enzymes metabolize neurotransmitters and limit the transport of these substances into brain. L-Dopa decarboxylase metabolizes L-dopa, reducing the amount of circulating L-dopa that can enter brain. An inhibitor of dopa decarboxylase, called carbidopa, is added to L-dopa for the treatment of Parkinson's disease by dopamine replacement. Polarity of enzymes appears to be important in function. The ATPase is located on the abluminal surface, where it is active in the secretion of interstitial fluid by creating a small osmotic imbalance when 3 molecules of Na^+ are exchanged for 2 molecules of K^+ (Betz and Goldstein, 1978). The mitochondria in endothelial cells are needed for generation of ATP. Lack of oxygen in ischemia and hypoxia interferes with this metabolic activity. Enzymes also are present to metabolize peptides and prevent their entry into brain.

7.2 GLUCOSE TRANSPORT

Glucose is carried into the brain by facilitated transport (Crone, 1965). When the concentration of glucose in the blood is low, it is more avidly transported across the capillary by the carrier mechanism. However, high concentrations of the glucose saturate the carrier molecules, and only a limited amount of glucose enters the brain by diffusion. The transport process is described by equations derived from enzyme kinetics, with the carrier molecule acting as the enzyme that causes the reaction to occur but remains unchanged in the process. Carrier molecules specifically transport D-glucose rather than L-glucose.

Analysis of glucose movement across the capillary is complicated because glucose is both transported and metabolized. To overcome this limitation analogs of glucose have been used. One such analog, 3-0-methylglucose is transported by the D-glucose carrier but is not metabolized by the tricarboxylic acid (TCA) cycle; it is a measure of glucose uptake (Pardridge and

Table 7–1. Enzymes and Transport Molecules in Cerebral Capillaries

Enzyme	Function	References
Dopa-decarboxylase	Metabolizes L-dopa	Bjorklund et al., 1969
Gamma-glutamyltranspeptidase	Metabolizes peptides	Albert et al., 1966
Na^+,K^+-ATPase	Active exchange of K and Na at cell membrane	Firth, 1977
Adenylate cyclase	Forms cAMP	Joo, 1975
Glucose transporter	Transports glucose into brain	Lidinsky and Drewes, 1983

Derived from Bradbury, 1984.

Oldendorf, 1975). Another analog of glucose, 2-deoxyglucose, is transported and phosphorylated but not further metabolized and is used to study the initial steps of glucose utilization (Sokoloff, 1981a). Analogs of glucose labeled with positron emitting isotopes have been used recently in PET scanning to measure glucose metabolism.

Transport of glucose in humans has been monitored using ^{11}C-3-0-methyl-D-glucose (^{11}C-MeG). The MeG competes with D-glucose for carrier-mediated transport. It is taken up by brain but not metabolized. If cerebral blood flow is measured simultaneously, it is possible to compute regional ^{11}C-MeG extraction. Use of ^{11}C-MeG for glucose transport requires three rate constants to fit the data. This suggests that, in addition to movement into and out of the brain, there may be uptake by a slow brain compartment (Brooks et al., 1986).

Glucose is transported across both sides of the endothelial cell and back into the blood (Figure 7–3). Glucose concentration in the plasma affects the transport rate between the plasma and intracellular compartment because of carrier-mediated transport. The transport constant term is K_m^T. Once within the cell, the concentration of glucose, C_s, affects the formation of metabolic products, C_p, and the metabolic processes are described by K_m^m. As the plasma concentration of glucose increases, the rate of influx becomes saturated, to reach a maximum where additional glucose enters by diffusion (Figure 7–4). Normal plasma levels are close to the estimated K_m^T, or Michaelis-Menten constant for half maximum influx. After entering the cell, glucose is metabolized through glycolysis and the Krebs cycle.

The relationship of glucose transport (supply) to glycolysis (demand) is determined from the concentrations of the substrates and K_m^T. For glucose, the transport step involves molecular movement across the endothelial cell, through the extracellular space, and into the cell. The K_m^T for transport is normally 6–10 μmol ml^{-1}, which is close to the normal value of glucose in the plasma (7–8 μmol ml^{-1}). Therefore, when blood glucose levels are low, as in hypoglycemia, metabolism is decreased because of decreased supply. High glucose plasma levels shift the rate-limiting step into the cell to the phosphorylation step. Table 7–2 is a comparison of glucose transport characteristics in brain, muscle, and liver. When the concentration of glucose in plasma is in the normal range, the transport system for brain is close

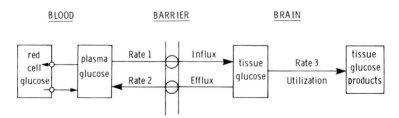

Figure 7–3. Transport steps in glucose entry into cells. Transfer from blood to cells involves movement across both membranes of the barrier, diffusion into brain, and utilization. (From Cremer et al., 1986)

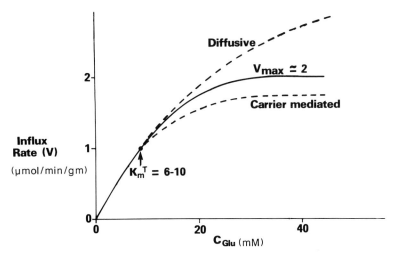

Figure 7–4. Schematic diagram of glucose transport into brain (V) plotted against arterial glucose concentration, C_{Glu}. The Michaelis-Menten transfer constant K_m^T and the V_{max} at saturation of the carrier are given. The normal glucose concentration in plasma is close to the K_m for transport.

to saturation, and transport rather than phosphorylation through hexokinase is rate-limiting. This situation is not present in liver, where glucokinase limits the metabolism of glucose.

Cremer et al. (1983) have calculated the rate of glucose transport and metabolism in the visual cortex of the awake rat. They found that as the cerebral blood volume increases, there is a linear increase in the transport maximum. This appears to be due to the recruitment of capillaries, with an increase in the available surface area. There are similarities in the rate of glucose transport between the rat and humans (Table 7–3).

7.3 DEOXYGLUCOSE AUTORADIOGRAPHY

Sokoloff et al. (1977) have developed a method to follow glucose transport into brain from blood and its incorporation into the metabolic cycle (Figure 7–5). The basis of the method is that 2-deoxyglucose (2-DG) is transported

Table 7–2. Comparison of Glucose Metabolism in Brain, Muscle, and Liver

	Brain	Muscle	Liver
Intracellular concentration	2–3 μmol/g	Very low	High
Enzyme (K_m^m)	Hexokinase (K_m = 8–30 μm)	Hexokinase	Glucokinase (K_m = 12–33 μm)
Limiting step	Transport into brain	Transport into muscle	Phosphorylation

Table 7–3. Average Values for Glucose Supply and Utilization in Human and Rat Brain

	Human	Rat
Blood glucose (mM)	6	6
Cerebral blood flow (ml g^{-1} min^{-1})	0.5	1.0
Supply of glucose to brain (μmol g^{-1} min^{-1})	3.0	6.0
Fractional glucose extraction by brain	0.1	0.13

Data from Cremer, 1986.

similarly to glucose across the blood–brain barrier. However, once within the cell, it is metabolized only up to the phosphorylation step. Quantitative autoradiography is done with 2-deoxy-D-^{14}C-glucose (^{14}C-DG). The ^{14}C-labeled compound is injected, and after 30–45 minutes has elapsed to allow uptake of all the substrate, the brain is removed, and autoradiograms are

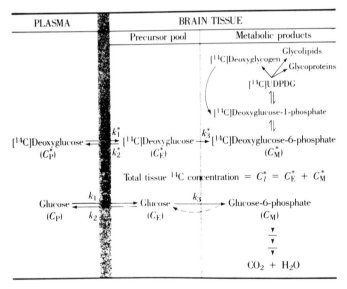

Figure 7–5. Diagrammatic representation of the theoretical 2-deoxyglucose model. C* represents the total ^{14}C concentration in a single homogeneous tissue of the brain. C_P^* and C_P represent the concentrations of ^{14}C-deoxyglucose and glucose in the arterial plasma, respectively. C_E^* and C_E represent their respective concentrations in the tissue pools that serve as substrates for hexokinase. C_M^* represents the concentration of ^{14}C-deoxyglucose-6-phosphate in the tissue. The constants k_1^*, k_2^*, and k_3^* represent the rate constants for carrier-mediated transport of ^{14}C-deoxyglucose from plasma to tissue, for carrier-mediated transport back from tissue to plasma, and for phosphorylation by hexokinase, respectively. The constants k_1, k_2, and k_3 are the equivalent rate constants for glucose. ^{14}C-deoxyglucose and glucose share and compete for the carrier that transports both between plasma and tissue and for hexokinase, which phosphorylates them to their respective hexose-6-phosphates. The dashed arrow represents the possibility of glucose-6-phosphate hydrolysis by glucose-6-phosphatase activity. (From Sokoloff et al., 1977)

prepared. With knowledge of the final concentration in the brain and the history of the isotope in the blood, an estimate of cerebral metabolic rate for glucose is obtainable (Figure 7–6).

In order to solve for the glucose metabolic rate, a lumped parameter is determined (Table 7–4). This parameter is determined for different species, regions, and disease states. However, assumptions about the lumped parameter may limit its usefulness in pathological situations. The assumptions made in the use of the 2-DG method are that the 2-DG is transported in both directions between blood and brain by the glucose transporter, that it is phosphorylated by hexokinase to deoxyglucose-6-phosphate (DG-6-P) and that it is trapped in the phosphate form for a sufficiently long period of time to prevent its loss from the brain while the 2-DG procedure is performed. The last assumption is critical, since the metabolism of DG-6-P would result in an underestimate of the amount in the brain and of the metabolic rate. Determination of the lumped parameter has been made for individual regions and in both conscious and anesthetized rats (Sokoloff, 1981a).

GENERAL EQUATION
FOR MEASUREMENT OF REACTION RATES WITH TRACERS:

$$\text{Rate of reaction} = \frac{\text{Labeled product formed in interval of time, 0 to } T}{\left[\begin{array}{c}\text{Isotope effect}\\ \text{correction factor}\end{array}\right]\left[\begin{array}{c}\text{Integrated specific activity}\\ \text{of precursor}\end{array}\right]}$$

OPERATIONAL EQUATION OF [^{14}C] DEOXYGLUCOSE METHOD:

Labeled product formed in interval of time, 0 to T

$$R_i = \frac{\overbrace{C_i^*(T)}^{\substack{\text{Total }^{14}\text{C in tissue}\\ \text{at time } T}} - \overbrace{k_1^* \, e^{-(k_2^* + k_3^*)T}\int_0^T C_P^* \, e^{(k_2^* + k_3^*)t}dt}^{\substack{^{14}\text{C in precursor remaining in tissue}\\ \text{at time } T}}}{\underbrace{\left[\frac{\lambda \cdot V_m^* \cdot K_m}{\Phi \cdot V_m \cdot K_m^*}\right]}_{\substack{\text{"Isotope effect"}\\ \text{correction factor}}}\underbrace{\left[\underbrace{\int_0^T \left(\frac{C_P^*}{C_P}\right)dt}_{\substack{\text{Integrated plasma}\\ \text{specific activity}}} - \underbrace{e^{-(k_2^* + k_3^*)T}\int_0^T \left(\frac{C_P^*}{C_P}\right)e^{(k_2^* + k_3^*)t}dt}_{\substack{\text{Correction for lag in tissue}\\ \text{equilibration with plasma}}}\right]}_{\text{Integrated precursor specific activity in tissue}}}$$

Figure 7–6. Operational equation of radioactive deoxyglucose method and its functional anatomy. T represents the time at the termination of the experimental period: λ equals the ratio of the distribution space of deoxyglucose in the tissue to that of glucose, Φ equals the fraction of glucose that, once phosphorylated, continued down the glycolytic pathway, and K_m^*, V_m^*, K_m, and V_m represent the Michaelis-Menten kinetic constants of hexokinase for deoxyglucose and glucose, respectively. The other symbols are the same as those defined in Figure 7–5. (From Sokoloff, 1977)

Table 7–4. Values of the Lumped Constant in Several Species

Animal	Number of Animals	Mean ± SEM
Rat (conscious)	15	0.464 ± 0.026
Monkey (conscious)	7	0.344 ± 0.036
Cat (anesthetized)	6	0.411 ± 0.005
Dog (conscious)	7	0.558 ± 0.031
Sheep	5	0.416 ± 0.014

Data from Sokoloff et al., 1977 and Sokoloff, 1981a.

The assumption of DG-6-P constancy has been disputed by studies that have shown a slow loss of the substrate from brain (Huang and Veech, 1985). It is debatable whether the rate of loss is great enough to interfere with measurement of glucose metabolism. This limitation can be overcome by two methods: (1) by incorporation of a term for metabolism of DG-6-P into the equations or (2) by use of a different tracer. Another potential tracer for use in glucose metabolism studies is radiolabeled glucose. Glucose labeled in the 1 or 2 position is rapidly converted into CO_2 (Hawkins et al., 1985). However, by labeling it in the 6 position, it remains within brain for a sufficiently long period to allow it to be studied. Regional metabolic rates for glucose have been compared using either $6\text{-}^{14}C$-glucose or $2\text{-}^{14}C$-deoxy-D-glucose (Hawkins et al., 1988). The glucose-infused animals were killed 5 minutes after injection, and the 2-DG-infused animals were killed after 45 minutes. Glucose metabolic rate was found to be higher in the glucose animals, and a slow loss of DG-6-P was suggested as the cause of the discrepancy. Corrections can be made in the operational 2-DG equations to account for the loss of DG-6-P. A comparison with PET scanning of the metabolic rate for glucose using ^{11}C-labeled glucose and DG showed a lower rate for the glucose-labeled compound, probably due to the loss of CO_2 from the glucose labeled in the 2 position (Stone-Elander et al., 1985). Studies with glucose labeled in the 6 position have not been reported for PET.

Metabolic activity has been studied by the 2-DG method under numerous conditions. In early studies using the method, it was found that the auditory system normally has a very high metabolic rate, deeper midline structures have moderate rates, and white matter has a very low rate (Sokoloff et al., 1977). Extensive studies on the visual system have been done with the 2-DG method. Kennedy et al. (1976) showed interdigitation of the visual cortex in animals with monocular occlusion (Figure 7–7). Numerous pathological conditions have been studied using the 2-DG method.

Blood flow is tightly coupled to brain function in most situations (Sokoloff, 1981b; Lou et al.; 1987). The basis of the coupling is debated. There are a number of vasoactive substances that are produced during metabolism, including acetylcholine, dopamine, norepinephrine, serotonin, adenosine, and a number of neuropeptides. Other factors active in the control of cerebral blood flow are arterial P_{CO_2}, pH, P_{O_2}. Under some circumstances the relationship of flow to metabolism breaks down, as in bicuculline seizures where flow increases out of proportion to metabolism. There are brainstem

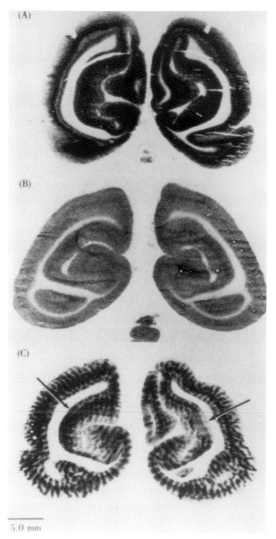

5.0 mm

Figure 7–7. Autoradiographs of coronal brain sections from rhesus monkeys at the level of the striate cortex. A. Animal with normal binocular vision. Note the laminar distribution of the density; the dark band corresponds to layer IV. B. Animal with bilateral visual deprivation. Note the almost uniform and reduced relative density, especially the virtual disappearance of the dark band corresponding to layer IV. C. Animal with right eye occluded. The half-brain on the left of the photograph represents the left hemisphere contralateral to the occluded eye. Note the alternate dark and light striations (each approximately 0.3–0.4 mm in width) that represent the ocular dominance columns. These columns are most apparent in the dark band corresponding to layer IV, but they extend through the entire thickness of the cortex. The arrows point to regions of bilateral asymmetry, where the ocular dominance columns are absent. These are presumably areas that normally receive only monocular input. The one on the left, contralateral to the occluded eye, has a continuous dark lamina corresponding to layer IV, which is completely absent on the side ipsilateral to the occluded representations of the blind spots. (From Kennedy et al., 1976)

129

mechanisms that regulate blood flow. Stimulation of dorsal medullary reticular formation results in an increase in regional blood flow (Iadecola et
al., 1983).

7.4 BLOOD–BRAIN BARRIER TRANSPORT BY AUTORADIOGRAPHY

Autoradiography has been adapted to analyze blood–brain barrier transport
of ^{14}C-labeled aminoisobutyric acid (AIB) (Blasberg et al., 1980). This compound is taken up slowly by cells, so that its content in brain is an indication
of the blood–brain transfer rate. For short periods of time, the transfer can
be modeled as one compartment. The AIB in brain (^{14}C-AIB)$_{br}$, the concentration in blood, C_{bl}, and the integral of the blood concentration over
time, T, are used to calculate the transfer rate, K.

$$K = \frac{(^{14}C\text{-AIB})_{br}}{\displaystyle\int_{o}^{T} C_{bl}dt} \tag{7–1}$$

This method has been used to measure uptake in several experimental pathological situations.

7.5 AMINO ACID TRANSPORT

Amino acids are abundant in the brain (Lajtha et al., 1981). The excitatory
amino acids, glutamate and aspartate, are found in high concentrations. Important neurotransmitter amino acids found in lower concentrations are glycine and γ-aminobutyric acid (GABA). Other brain amino acids are L-dopa,
leucine, phenylalanine, tryptophan, methionine, histidine, and valine. The
essential amino acids are required by brain for protein synthesis and neurotransmission. To ensure the uptake of the essential amino acids into brain,
carrier systems are found in the capillaries for their transport.

Carrier systems transport neutral amino acids, basic amino acids, and acidic
amino acids (Lajtha, 1974). Neutral amino acids are carried by the L-system
(leucine-preferring). Competitive inhibition of the L-system carrier prevents
the entry of essential amino acids in the presence of an excess of one of the
transported molecules. In the hereditary disorder in which an excess of phenylalanine is present in the blood, competition for the L carrier blocks the
entry of tryptophan, and serotonin levels in the brain are reduced by the
absence of its precursor, tryptophan. Individuals with increased phenylalanine in the blood have mental retardation, which can be prevented with a
diet low in phenylalanine (Pardridge and Choi, 1986).

The A-system, which carries α-(methylamino) isobutyric acid into cells
appears to be absent from brain tissue. Glycine enters brain slowly as does
glutamate, N-acetylaspartate, and aspartate. Efflux from brain appears to

occur actively for the acidic amino acids, glutamate, and aspartate (Pardridge and Choi, 1986). Utilization of amino acids is determined by the rate of their transport across the capillary and the amount of enzyme available in the cell. The amino acids have a low transport rate into the brain and a high enzymatic utilization rate. Therefore, the rate-limiting step is the passage into the brain. Kinetic transport constants are in the range of the serum concentrations for the amino acids. Inhibition of transport is thus possible. If the kinetic constants were high and enzyme utilization rates low, the amino acids could be transported easily into the brain, and an excess of one amino acid in the serum would not competitively inhibit the entrance of another. Compared to glucose, the rate of entry of the amino acids into brain is slow (Table 7–5).

The nonessential amino acids, glutamate and aspartate, are excitatory transmitters in the CNS. Glutamate and aspartate are incorporated into proteins and peptides, and glutamate also is essential in ammonia regulation.

Glutamate concentration in brain is 13.6 μmol/g as compared with 4.4 μmol/g for glutamine, 2.3 μmol/g for GABA, and 0.4 μmol/g of lysine. Although glutamate levels are high, it is compartmentalized, and only a portion is involved in neurotransmission. Glutamate is important in ammonia metabolism, since when ammonia levels are increased, as in hepatic disease, the ammonia is detoxified by conversion to glutamine, which is elevated in CSF and brain.

Essential amino acids are maintained in brain at levels close to those in plasma. Competitive inhibition interferes with transport of essential amino acids. Tyrosine, for example, moves into brain across cerebral capillaries by a carrier-mediated transport system. When amino acids using the same carrier are increased, the amount of tyrosine entering brain is reduced. Normally, tyrosine is converted by cells in the substantia nigra into dopamine. In patients with Parkinson's disease, the dopamine-forming cells of the substantia nigra are damaged, and L-dopa is taken orally in order to replace levels of brain dopamine. Large doses of L-dopa are needed to overcome the metabolic loss caused by the enzyme dopa decarboxylase in the blood

Table 7–5. Kinetic Constants of Blood–Brain Barrier Amino Acid and Monocarboxylic Acid Transport in Rat

	Substrate	K_m (μmol/ml)	V_{max} (μmol/min/gm)
Neutral amino acids	Leucine	.10	.022
	Phenylalanine	.11	.028
	L-Dopa	.43	.063
Basic amino acids	Arginine	.088	.008
	Lysine	.11	.008
Monocarboxylic acid	Lactic acid	1.8	.091
	Beta-hydroxybutyric acid	2.5	.16
Hexose	D-Glucose	7	1.5

Data from Pardridge, 1981, and Crone, 1986.

vessels. Carbidopa inhibits dopa decarboxylase, so that smaller doses of L-dopa can be used. Tyrosine and L-dopa uptake can be competitively inhibited by the presence of other amino acids after ingestion of protein.

7.6 GLUCOSE AND AMINO ACID METABOLISM

Brain glucose is metabolized to produce energy for cellular work or converted to amino acids and lipids (Gaitonde et al., 1965; Lehninger, 1971). The major pathway of energy production from glucose is the TCA cycle. Glucose is transported into the cell, where it undergoes glycolysis (Figure 7–8). The glucose molecule is phosphorylated by hexokinase into glucose

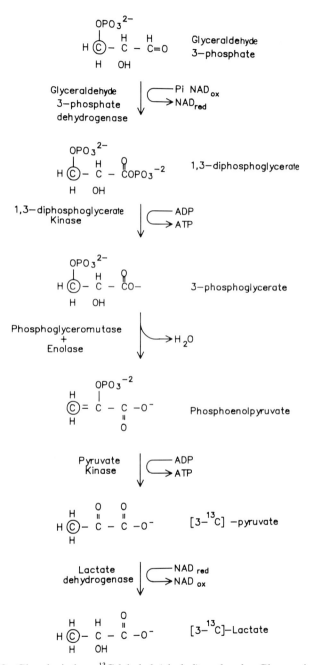

Figure 7–8. Glycolysis in a ^{13}C-labeled (circled) molecule. Glucose is labeled in the 1 position with ^{13}C. The products of glycolysis are 3-^{13}C-pyruvate and 3-^{13}C-lactate (Derived from Lehninger, 1971).

6-phosphate before conversion by phosphofructokinase into fructose 1,6-di-phosphate. Then it is split into glyceraldehyde 3-phosphate and dihydrox-yacetone phosphate. The rate-limiting enzyme is the ATP-sensitive phos-phofructokinase, which is inhibited by ATP, PCr, and citrate and activated by ADP, P_i, AMP, cyclic 3,5-AMP, and NH_4^+. The final products of gly-colysis are pyruvate and lactate.

Analysis of the TCA cycle has been done with ^{14}C-labeled substrates. Radioactively labeled molecules show the total concentration of metabolic products but require chemical separations for full characterization of the me-tabolites. Enrichment of a molecule with a ^{13}C label has the advantage of characterizing both the metabolic products and the exact position of the label in the metabolite. Use of ^{13}C labeling with NMR spectroscopy often can reduce the need for cumbersome chemical extractions. Thus, ^{13}C labeling and NMR provide a means to follow and characterize completely the passage of a labeled substrate through the TCA cycle. A glucose molecule labeled with ^{13}C in the 1 position becomes lactate labeled in the 3 position (Figure 7–9). In the mitochondria, pyruvate is decarboxylated to acetyl-CoA, which enters the Krebs cycle (Figure 6–14).

The Krebs cycle is crucial for production of NADH needed to replenish ATP. Acetyl-CoA also is formed by fatty acid oxidation and amino acid breakdown. Acetyl-CoA enters the cycle by forming citric acid after joining with oxaloacetate. Succeeding steps of metabolism convert citrate into al-pha-ketoglutaric acid, succinic acid, fumaric acid, malic acid, and finally back to oxaloacetic acid, completing the cycle. Alpha-ketoglutaric acid is metabolized to glutamic acid in the brain. One turn of the Krebs cycle makes 3 mol of reduced NAD. The NADH releases energy in the respiratory chain as electrons flow from it to oxygen.

$$\text{NADH} + 1/2\,O_2 + H^+ \rightarrow \text{NAD} + H_2O \qquad (7\text{--}2)$$

From glycolysis of glucose to pyruvate, there are 2 mol of ATP formed.

$$\text{Glucose} + 2\,\text{NAD} + 2\,\text{ADP} + 2\,P_i$$
$$\rightarrow 2\,\text{pyruvate} + 2\,\text{NADH} + 2\,H_2O + 2\,\text{ATP} \quad (7\text{--}3)$$

Each NADH molecule that is formed outside the mitochondria and metab-olized inside yields 2 ATP because of the loss of reducing potential during transport. Thus

$$2\,\text{NADH} + 4\,P_i + 4\,\text{ADP} + O_2 \rightarrow 2\,\text{NAD} + 6\,H_2O + 4\,\text{ATP} \quad (7\text{--}4)$$

Formation of 2 acetyl-CoA from 2 pyruvate inside the mitochondria yields 6 mol of ATP.

$$2\,\text{Pyruvate} + 2\,\text{NADCoA} \rightarrow 2\,\text{acetyl-CoA} + 2\,CO_2 + 2\,\text{NADH} \quad (7\text{--}5)$$
$$2\,\text{NADH} + 6\,P_i + 6\,\text{ADP} + O_2 \rightarrow 2\,\text{NAD} + 8\,H_2O + 6\,\text{ATP} \qquad (7\text{--}6)$$

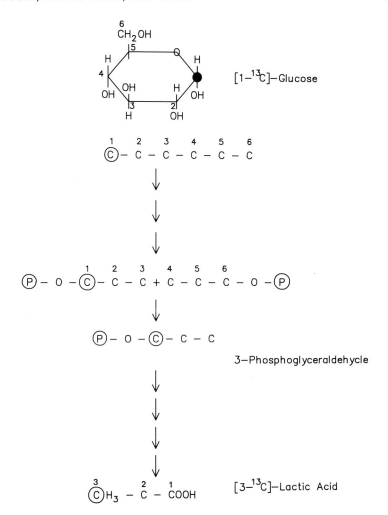

Figure 7–9. The pathway of carbon atoms in glycolysis. Glucose labeled in the 1 position with ^{13}C is found in the 3 position of lactate. Note that the numbering of the labeled carbon is determined by the position of the carboxyl group and that the numbering changes in the final product (Derived from Lehninger, 1971).

Finally, as 2 molecules of acetate go through the Krebs cycle and the respiratory chain, additional ATP is formed.

$$2 \text{ Acetyl CoA} + 24 \text{ P}_i + 24 \text{ ADP} + 4 O_2$$
$$\rightarrow 4 CO_2 + 28 H_2O + 24 \text{ ATP} \quad (7\text{–}7)$$

The energy yield from the complete metabolism of glucose is given by

$$\text{Glucose} + 36 \text{ P}_i + 36 \text{ ADP} + 6 O_2 \rightarrow 6 CO_2 + 42 H_2O + 36 \text{ ATP} \quad (7\text{–}8)$$

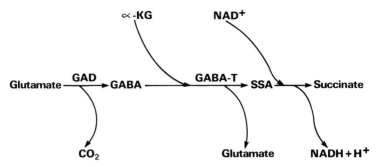

Figure 7–10. GABA shunt. Glutamate is converted to GABA and CO_2 by gluta-mate decarboxylase (GAD). GABA and alpha-ketoglutarate (α-KG) form succinate semialdehyde (SSA) and glutamate by GABA-transaminase (GABA-T). SSA is changed into succinate by SSA dehydrogenase. NAD is reduced to NADH by the reaction.

Therefore, the transfer of energy from glucose to ATP is a highly efficient process that effectively allows the intact cell to burn glucose into calories for use and storage rather than for generation of heat.

7.7 AMINO ACID NEUROTRANSMITTERS

Glutamate is the main excitatory neurotransmitter substance, and GABA is the major inhibitory transmitter in brain. The enzymes involved in gluta-mate–GABA metabolism are listed in Table 7–6. GABA is formed irrevers-ibly from glutamate via the enzyme glutamic acid decarboxylase (GAD). Once formed, GABA is released as a neurotransmitter at the synapse. Reup-take occurs either into the neuron or into the astrocyte, where GABA-trans-aminase (GABA-T) and a dehydrogenase return it to the TCA cycle as suc-cinate. The return of GABA to the TCA cycle is referred to as the GABA shunt (Figure 7–10). The enzymes GABA-T and succinic semialdehyde de-hydrogenase (SSADH) are located in the mitochondria. Nerve cell endings contain the enzyme GAD in the cytosol (Ribak et al., 1977). Glial cells lack GAD; they can convert glutamate via glutamine synthetase into glutamine

Table 7–6. Enzymes Involved in Glutamate and GABA Metabolism

Enzyme	Action
Glutamate oxaloacetate aminotransferase (GOT)	Transamination between glutamate/alpha-ketoglutarate and aspartate/oxaloacetate
Glutamine synthetase (GLU-S)	Glutamine synthesis from glutamate and ammonia (ATP needed)
Glutamic acid decarboxylase (GAD)	GABA formation from glutamate
GABA transaminase (GABA-T)	GABA metabolized to succinate semialdehyde
Glutaminase (GLU-N)	Converts glutamine into glutamate

(Figure 7–11). Alpha-ketoglutarate available from the Krebs cycle is converted into glutamate by GABA-T in the mitochondria.

Compartments of glutamate are present in the brain (Lajtha et al., 1959; Berl et al., 1961). ^{14}C-glucose is mainly metabolized to glutamate, whereas ^{14}C-acetate is metabolized into glutamine. These studies led to the concept of two pools of glutamate, one for energy generation and another that gives rise to neurotransmitters (Van den Berg and Garfinkel, 1971). Glucose and pyruvate enter both pools, whereas acetate, acetaldelyde, propionate, butyrate, citrate, GABA, glutamate, aspartate, leucine, bicarbonate, ammonia, and succinate enter the small pool (Hertz, 1979). A model has been proposed in which the GAD-containing neurons make GABA from glutamate for use in neurotransmission, whereas its catabolism occurs via the GABA shunt in the astrocytes, where it is converted by GABA-T into glutamate and by glutamine synthetase into glutamine. The glutamine is then transported to the neuron for reconversion into GABA (Figure 7–11).

^{13}C-NMR studies of glucose, glutamate, and GABA metabolism have been performed to further elucidate their interactions (Brainard et al., 1989). Following injection of 1-^{13}C-glucose into pentobarbital-anesthetized rat, it is converted to 4-^{13}C-glutamate in the TCA cycle by the action of pyruvate dehydrogenase (Figure 6–14). Ninety percent of the labeled glucose appears in 4-^{13}C-glutamate via pyruvate dehydrogenase, whereas 10 percent is metabolized by pyruvate carboxylase to 2-^{13}C-glutamate (Figure 7–12). The metabolism of 1-^{13}C-glucose by pyruvate carboxylase occurs by the ana-

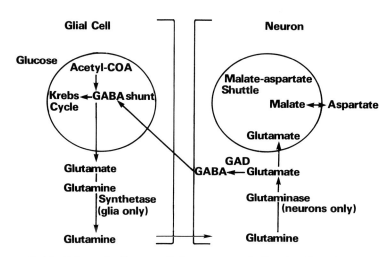

Figure 7–11. Schematic diagram of glutamate metabolism in glia and neurons. Circled area is mitochondria. Glucose enters the GABA shunt as acetyl-COA. Glutamate in the glial cell cytosol is converted to glutamine by glutamine synthetase present only in glia. Glutamine enters the neuron, where it is converted to glutamate by glutaminase. GAD converts glutamate to GABA, which goes into the GABA shunt in the gial cell, or glutamate is incorporated into the malate–aspartate shuttle in the mitochondria of the neuron. (Based on Benjamin and Quastel, 1975)

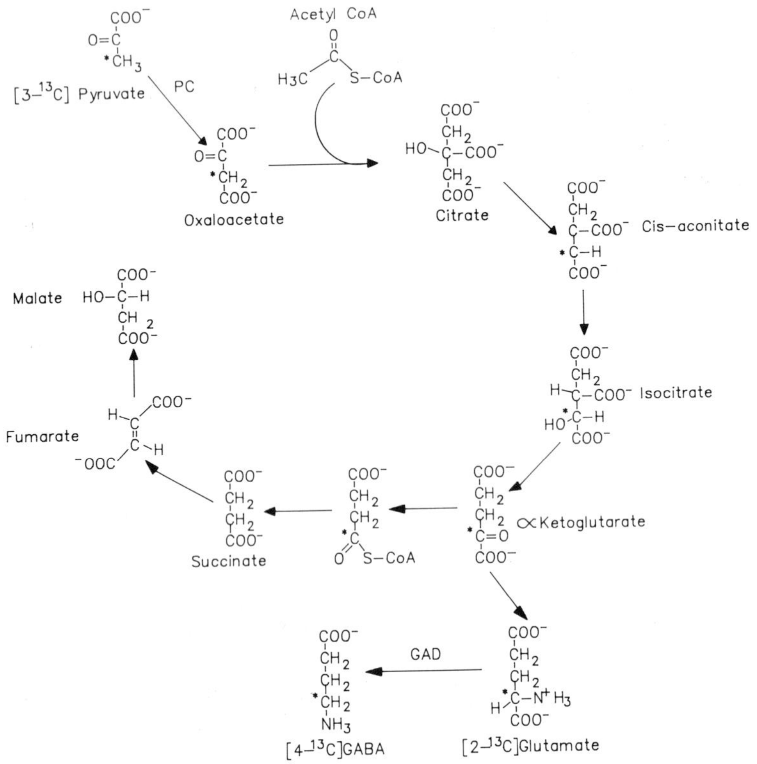

Figure 7–12. The TCA cycle is shown for metabolism of 1-^{13}C-glucose via pyruvate carboxylase (PC). Glutamate labeled in the second position is converted to GABA labeled in the fourth position by GAD. The convention for labeling is to count the carbon closest to the carboxyl group (or with the most nonproton bonds) as the first carbon.

plerotic reaction in which oxaloacetate is formed. The ^{13}C label, therefore, is in the second carbon of glutamate and the fourth carbon of GABA. The location of the ^{13}C in GABA indicates the metabolic pathway followed. For example, 4-^{13}C-GABA is a product of pyruvate carboxylase, and 2-^{13}C-GABA formed from 4-^{13}C-glutamate is a product of pyruvate dehydrogenase.

The morphological basis of the current model of glutamate–glutamine interaction is controversial. Problems with isolation of pure fractions and possible differences between species have complicated the interpretation of data. A major problem with the current model is the slow uptake of glutamine by neurons, which is important in the conversion of glutamine to glutamate in the neuron. Although there is general agreement that an anaplerotic reaction with carbon fixation by pyruvate carboxylase exists in brain and accounts for about 10 percent of glucose metabolism (Patel, 1974), the location of this enzyme is controversial. A model has been proposed in which the pyruvate carboxylase participates in an incomplete TCA cycle (Hertz, 1979).

This model is consistent with the ^{13}C-glucose biochemical data in rats (Figure 7–13).

Immunohistochemical studies, however, suggest that pyruvate carboxylase is in the astrocyte in the same compartment with glutamine synthetase (Shank and Campbell, 1984; Yu et al., 1983). At present, there is no model that will explain both the biochemical and the histological data. The carboxylation of pyruvate to oxaloacetate appears to occur within the small biosynthetic compartment, whereas the conversion of glucose to glutamate by pyruvate dehydrogenase is in another compartment. What molecule shuttles between the two compartments and whether they cross cell types, however, remain to be determined.

7.8 LIPID METABOLISM

Brain tissue has a high content of lipids. Cholesterol, sphingolipids, and glycerophospholipids comprise the three major categories of brain lipids (Suzuki, 1981). Cholesterol is important in membrane structure for all cells, including those of brain tissue. Sphingolipids are important components of the myelin sheath. Glycerophospholipids are important in membrane structure and in lipid metabolism, since they play a role in normal metabolism and release substances that lead to cellular disruption.

Glycerophospholipids are formed around the glycerol backbone. Two long-chain fatty acids are present, along with a phosphate-linked substance from which the molecule derives its name. Figure 7–14 shows the basic structure of the phosphatidyl moiety. One compound in brain is phosphatidylethanolamine. When the substitution at A is inositol with or without additional phosphates the compound is termed phosphatidylinositol (PI). Breakdown of PI occurs primarily by phospholipase C and A_2 (Figure 7–15).

The long-chain fatty acids at position 1 are oriented in the hydrocarbon part of the membrane, whereas those at position 2 are in the water–hydro-

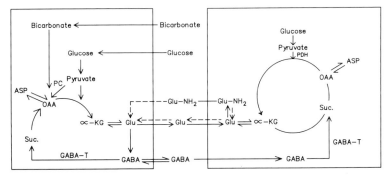

Figure 7–13. An alternative hypothetical model of glutamate–GABA metabolism based on two compartments. Solid lines represent dominant direction. (Modified from Hertz, 1979)

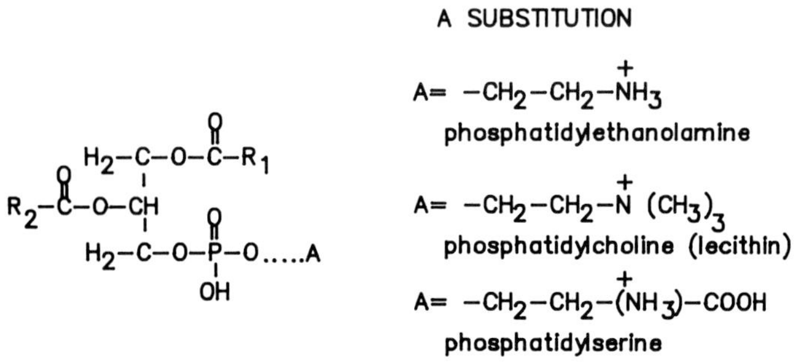

A SUBSTITUTION

$$A= -CH_2-CH_2-\overset{+}{N}H_3$$
phosphatidylethanolamine

$$A= -CH_2-CH_2-\overset{+}{N} (CH_3)_3$$
phosphatidylcholine (lecithin)

$$A= -CH_2-CH_2-\overset{+}{(NH_3)}-COOH$$
phosphatidylserine

Figure 7–14. The basic structure of a phospholipid is shown. The glycerol molecule is the backbone to which fatty acids are attached at R_1 and R_2. The phosphate links the various molecules shown as substitutions at A.

carbon interface. Snake venom and pancreatic enzymes contain large amounts of phospholipase A_2 in a soluble, easily extractable form, making it convenient to study. Trypsin activates the enzyme. However, there is phospholipase associated with membranes. Phospholipase A_2 has been purified from rat liver mitochondria, where it is bound to membranes and present in low concentrations that are in continuous contact with an excess of substrate (De Winter et al., 1982). When respiration of the mitochondria is reduced, the enzyme is activated and hydrolyzes membranes (Parce et al., 1978).

Phospholipase C releases inositol from PI. It has been identified in brain, muscle, platelets, and seminal fluid. The enzyme is important in the PI cycle, where it hydrolyses PI into diacylglycerol (DAG) and inositol mono-, di-, and triphosphate. DAG activates protein kinase C and is a source of arachidonic acid.

Fatty acids are named by the length of their chains, a, and the number of

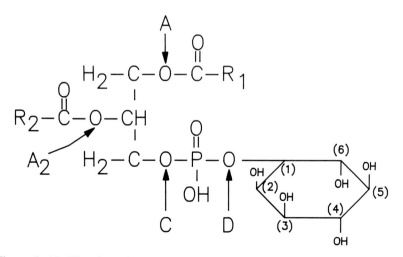

Figure 7–15. The sites of action of lipases on the phosphatidylinositol molecule.

unsaturated, double bonds, b (a:b). The commonly occurring fatty acids are palmitic (16:0), stearic (18:0), and arachidonic (20:4). Less commonly found in brain membranes are oleic (18:1) and linoleic acid (18:2). For example, PI contains 45.5 percent arachidonic acid, 34.4 percent stearic acid, 9.5 percent palmitic acid, 6.4 percent oleic acid, and 2.3 percent docosahexaenoic acid.

Phosphatidylethanolamine contains 12.5 percent arachidonic acid and 40.2 percent plasmalogen, and phosphatidylcholine has 46.9 percent palmitic acid and 6.0 percent arachidonic acid. This information is important in attempting to understand the mechanism of fatty acid release during brain injury. PI appears to play a central role in the release of arachidonic acid, which damages cells through its metabolic products.

Arachidonic acid is a C_{20} fatty acid that is the precursor of a group of molecules collectively termed the eicosanoids. These include prostaglandins, thromboxanes, leukotrienes, and hydroxyeicosanoic acids. The eicosanoids are formed by the action of cyclooxygenase and lipoxygenase in the presence of oxygen.

Arachidonic acid usually is found free in cells in concentrations of less that $10^{-6}M$. For the arachidonic cascade to begin, it is necessary to first remove the inositol group by the action of membrane-bound phospholipase C, leaving DAG. DAG is hydrolyzed to a monoglycerol by DG lipase, releasing stearic acid from position 1. Further enzymatic action releases arachidonic acid from position 2.

Normally the PI cycle is activated as part of the second messenger system of membranes (Michell et al., 1979; Berridge et al., 1984; Williamson et al., 1985). The arachidonic acid also is derived from the hydrolysis of phosphatidylcholine, where it is found in a small percentage of fatty acids, by the activation of phospholipases C and A_2. Molecules attach to receptors on the cell surface and activate the second messenger cascade. Protein kinase C is activated and initiates protein phosphorylation and calcium influx into the cytosol. This process is usually self-limiting and necessary in chemical signaling in the cell. However, at times, it becomes excessive, and the by-products, such as arachidonic acid and calcium, damage cells.

REFERENCES

Albert, Z., Orlowski, M., Rzucidlo, Z., Orlowska, J.: Studies on gamma-glutamyl transpeptidase activity and its histochemical localization in the central nervous system of man and different animal species. Acta. Histochem. (Jena) 25:312–320 1966.

Benjamin, A. M., Quastel, J. H.: Metabolism of amino acids and ammonia in rat brain cortex sites in vitro: A possible role of ammonia in brain. J. Neurochem. 25:197–206, 1975.

Berl, S., Lajtha, A., Waelch, H.: Amino acid and protein metabolism—VI. Cerebral compartments of glutamic acid metabolism. J. Neurochem. 7:186–197, 1961.

Berridge, M. J., Irvine, R. F.: Inositol trisphosphate, a novel second messenger in cellular signal transduction. Nature 312:315–321, 1984.

Betz, A. L., Goldstein, G. W.: Polarity of the blood–brain barrier: Neutral amino acid transport into isolated brain capillaries. Science 202:225–227, 1978.

Bjorklund, A., Falck, B., Hromek, F., Owman, C.: An enzymic barrier mechanism for monamine precursors in the newly forming brain capillaries following electrolytic or mechanical lesions. J. Neurochem. 16:1605–1608, 1969.

Blasberg, R. G., Gazendam, J., Patlak, C. S., Fenstermacher, J. D.: Quantitative autoradiographic studies of brain edema and a comparison of multi-isotope autoradiographic techniques. Adv. Neurol. 28:255–270, 1980.

Bradbury, M. W. B.: The Concept of a Blood–Brain Barrier. Chichester, England: John Wiley & Sons, 1979.

Bradbury, M. W. B.: The structure and function of the blood–brain barrier. Fed. Proc. 43:186–190, 1984.

Bradbury, M. W., Stulcova, B.: Efflux mechanism contributing to the stability of the potassium concentration in cerebrospinal fluid. J. Physiol. (Lond) 208:415–430, 1970.

Brainard, J. R., Kyner, E., Rosenberg, G. A.: ^{13}C NMR evidence for GABA formation via pyruvate carboxylase in rat brain: A metabolic basis for compartmentation. J. Neurochem. 53:1285–1292, 1989.

Brooks, D. J., Beaney, R. P., Lammertsma, A. A., Herold, S., Turton, D. R., Luthra, S. K., Frackowiak, R. S., Thomas, D. G., Marshall, J., Jones, T.: Glucose transport across the blood–brain barrier in normal human subjects and patients with cerebral tumours studied using [^{11}C]3-0-methyl-D-glucose and positron emission tomography. J. Cereb. Blood Flow Metab. 6:230–239, 1986.

Cremer, J. E.: In Blood–Brain Barrier in Health and Disease. Suckling, A. J., Rumsby, M. G., Bradbury, M. W. B., eds. Chichester, England: Ellis Horwood, 1986:73–86.

Cremer, J. E., Cunningham, V. J., Seville, M. P.: Relationships between extraction and metabolism of glucose, blood flow, and tissue blood volume in regions of rat brain. J. Cereb. Blood Flow Metab. 3:291–302, 1983.

Crone, C.: Facilitated transfer of glucose from blood into brain tissue. J. Physiol. (Lond) 181:103–113, 1965.

Crone, C.: The blood–brain barrier as a tight epithelium: Where is information lacking? Ann. NY Acad. Sci. 481:174–185, 1986.

Crone, C., Christensen, O.: Electrical resistance of a capillary endothelium. J. Gen. Physiol. 77:349–371, 1981.

Crone, C., Olesen, S. P.: Electrical resistance of brain microvascular endothelium. Brain Res. 241:49–55, 1982.

De Winter, J. M., Vianen, G. M., Van den Bosch, H.: Purification of rat liver mitochondrial phospholipase A_2. Biochim. Biophys. Acta. 712:332–341, 1982.

Firth, J. A.: Cytochemical localization of the K^+ regulation interface between blood and brain. Experientia 33:1093–1094, 1977.

Gaitonde, M. K., Dahl, D. R., Elliott, K. A. C.: Entry of glucose carbon into amino acids of rat brain and liver in vivo after injection of uniformly ^{14}C-labelled glucose. Biochem. J. 94:345–352, 1965.

Goldstein, G. W., Betz, A. L.: Recent advances in understanding brain capillary function. Ann. Neurol. 14:389–395, 1983.

Hawkins, R. A., Mans, A. M., Davis, D. W., DeJoseph, M. R.: Comparison of

[^{14}C]glucose and [^{14}C]deoxyglucose as tracers of brain glucose use. Am. J. Physiol. 254:E310–E317, 1988.

Hawkins, R. A., Mans, A. M., Davis, D. W., Vina, J. R., Hibbard, L. S.: Cerebral glucose use measured with [^{14}C]glucose labeled in the 1,2 or 6 position. Am. J. Physiol. 248:C170–C176, 1985.

Hertz, L.: Functional interactions between neurons and astrocytes I. Turnover and metabolism of putative amino acid transmitters. Prog. Neurobiol. 13:277–323, 1979.

Huang, M. T., Veech, R. L.: Metabolic fluxes between [^{14}C]-2-deoxy-D-glucose and [^{14}C]2-deoxy-D-glucose 6-phosphate in brain in vivo. J. Neurochem. 44:567–573, 1985.

Iadecola, C., Nakai, M., Arbit, E., Reis, D. J.: Global cerebral vasodilatation elicited by focal electrical stimulation within the dorsal medullary reticular formation in anesthetized rat. J. Cereb. Blood Flow Metab. 3:270–279, 1983.

Joo, F., Toth, I.: Brain adenylate cyclase: Its common occurrence in the capillaries and astrocytes. Naturwissenschaften 62:397–398, 1975.

Kennedy, C., Des Rosiers, M. H., Sakurada, O., Shinohara, M., Reivich, M., Jehle, J. W., Sokoloff, L.: Metabolic mapping of the primary visual system of the monkey by means of the autoradiographic [^{14}C]deoxyglucose technique. Proc. Natl. Acad. Sci. USA 73:4230–4234, 1976.

Lajtha, A.: In *Aromatic Amino Acids in the Brain*. Wolstenholme, G. E. W., Fitzsimons, D. W., eds. Amsterdam: Elsevier, 1974:25–41.

Lajtha, A., Berl, S., Waelsch, H.: Amino acids and protein metabolism of the brain— IV. The metabolism of glutamic acid. J. Neurochem. 3:322–332, 1959.

Lajtha, A. L., Maker, H. S., Clarke, D. D.: In *Basic Neurochemistry*. Siegel, G. J., Albers, R. W., Agranoff, B. W., Katzman, R., eds. Boston: Little, Brown and Company, 1981:329–353.

Lehninger, A. L.: *Bioenergetics*. Menlo Park, California: W. A. Benjamin, 1971.

Lidinsky, W. A., Drewes, L. R.: Characterization of the blood–brain barrier: Protein composition of the capillary endothelial cell membrane. J. Neurochem. 41:1341–1348, 1983.

Lou, H. C., Edvinsson, L., MacKenzie, E. T.: The concept of coupling blood flow to brain function: Revision required. Ann. Neurol. 22:289–297, 1987.

Michell, R. H., Kirk, C. J., Billah, M. M.: Hormonal stimulation of phosphatidylinositol breakdown with particular reference to the hepatic effects of vasopressin. Biochem. Soc. Trans. 7:861–865, 1979.

Parce, J. W., Cunningham, C. C., Waite, M.: Mitochondrial phospholipase A$_2$ activity and mitochondrial aging. Biochemistry 17:1634–1639, 1978.

Pardridge, W. M.: Brain metabolism: A perspective from the blood–brain barrier. Physiol. Rev. 63:1481–1535, 1983.

Pardridge, W. M., Choi, T. B.: Neutral amino acid transport at the human blood–brain barrier. Fed. Proc. 45:2073–2078, 1986.

Pardridge, W. M., Oldendorf, W. H.: Kinetics of blood–brain transport of hexoses. Biochim. Biophys. Acta. 382:377–392, 1975.

Patel, M. S.: The relative significance of CO_2-fixing enzymes in the metabolism of rat brain. J. Neurochem. 22:717–724, 1974.

Rapoport, S. I.: *The Blood–Brain Barrier in Physiology and Medicine*. New York: Raven Press, 1976.

Reese, I. S., Karnovsky, M. J.: Find structural localization of a blood–brain barrier to exogenous peroxidase. J. Cell Biol. 34:207–217, 1967.

Ribak, C. E., Vaughn, J. E., Saito, K., Barber, R., Roberts, E.: Glutamate decarboxylase localization in neurons of the olfactory bulb. Brain Res. 126:1–
   18, 1977.
Shank, R. P., Campbell, G. L.: Alpha-ketoglutarate and malate uptake and metabolism by synaptosomes: Further evidence for an astrocyte-to-neuron metabolic shuttle. J. Neurochem. 42:1153–1161, 1984.
Sokoloff, L.: Localization of functional activity in the central nervous system by
   measurement of glucose utilization with radioactive deoxyglucose. J. Cereb.
   Blood Flow Metab. 1:7–36, 1981.
Sokoloff, L.: Relationships among local functional activity, energy metabolism, and
   blood flow in the central nervous system. Fed. Proc. 40:2311–2316, 1981b.
Sokoloff, L., Reivich, M., Kennedy, C., Des Rosiers, M. H., Patlak, C. S., Pettigrew, K. D., Sakurada, O., Shinohara, M.: The [^{14}C]deoxyglucose method
   for the measurement of local cerebral glucose utilization: Theory, procedure,
   and normal values in the conscious and anesthetized albino rat. J. Neurochem. 28:897–916, 1977.
Stewart, P. A., Wiley, M. J.: Developing nervous tissue induces formation of blood–
   brain barrier characteristics in invading endothelial cells: A study using quail-
   chick transplantation chimeras. Dev. Biol. 84:183–192, 1981.
Stone-Elander, S., Nilsson, J. L. G., Blomqvist, G., Ehrin, E., Eriksson, L., Gar-
   melius, B., Greitz, T., Johnstrom, P., Sjogren, I., Widen, L.: ^{11}C-2-Deoxy-
   D-glucose: Synthesis and preliminary comparison with ^{11}C-D-Glucose as a
   tracer for cerebral energy metabolism in PET studies. Eur. J. Nucl. Med.
   10:481–486, 1985.
Suzuki, K.: In *Basic Neurochemistry*. Siegel, G. J., Albers, R. W., Agranoff, B.
   W., Katzman, R., eds. Boston: Little, Brown and Company, 1981:355–370.
Takasato, Y., Rapoport, S. I., Smith, Q. R.: An in situ brain perfusion technique
   to study cerebrovascular transport in the rat. Am. J. Physiol. 247:H484–H493,
   1984.
Van Den Berg, C. J., Garfinkel, D.: A stimulation study of brain compartments.
   Metabolism of glutamate and related substances in mouse brain. Biochem.
   J. 123:211–218, 1971.
Williamson, J. R., Cooper, R. H., Joseph, S. K., Thomas, A. P.: Inositol tris-
   phosphate and diacylglycerol and intracellular second messengers in liver.
   Am. J. Physiol. 248:C203–C216, 1985.
Yu, A. C., Drejer, J., Hertz, L., Schousboe, A.: Pyruvate carboxylase activity in
   primary cultures of astrocytes and neurons. J. Neurochem. 41:1484–1487,
   1983.

8

Hypoxia–Ischemia

8.1 INTRODUCTION

Brain cells require a constant supply of glucose and oxygen to maintain normal brain function. Interruption of either energy source interferes with normal metabolism and, if prolonged, leads to irreversible cell damage. Circumstances leading to acute cerebral dysfunction occur frequently in patients with stroke, cardiac arrest, cardiac arrhythmias, anoxia from multiple causes, and raised intracranial pressure that interferes with cerebral blood flow (CBF). Subacute causes of brain dysfunction from energy substrate failure include such conditions as carbon monoxide poisoning and hypoglycemia. Lack of oxygen and blood loss often occur together, since when blood flow is disrupted, oxygen delivery stops. The term "hypoxia–ischemia" is used to describe this type of brain damage. Hypoxia can occur alone, however, as in anesthetic accidents in which nitrogen is substituted for oxygen, cyanide poisoning, and severe anemia.

During hypoxia–ischemia, a cascade of metabolic events results from the changeover from aerobic to anaerobic metabolism. A complex series of changes is triggered: lactate builds up inside the cell, lowering brain pH, energy charge stored as ATP and phosphocreatinine (PCr) is depleted, GABA begins to increase, and free fatty acids rise. Ionic changes occur along with amino acid alterations; extracellular potassium increases, the amino acid excitatory neurotransmitters glutamate and aspartate are released, and calcium enters cells and initiates degradative processes that result in membrane breakdown. Cells are irreversibly damaged once the membranes are disrupted. Treatment is, therefore, aimed at preventing the series of changes that lead to irreversible cell death.

Until recently, there was little to be offered for treatment of brain hypoxia–ischemia. Patients with strokes were treated for their medical prob-

145

lems, but no treatments were available for the stroke itself. The brain lesions were highly resistant to therapy. Temporary measures, such as hyperosmolar treatment with glycerol or mannitol, were used. Steroids had been used to treat ischemic edema, but there was little experimental evidence to support their use, and they are no longer recommended. Rehabilitation was the mainstay of treatment once the acute phase of the illness had passed.

Diagnosis of the extent of brain damage can be determined from the clinical examination. Angiography is used in patients suspected of having an aneurysm, vascular malformation, vasculitis, or tumor. Lack of blood flow in a markedly edematous brain can be used as an angiographic sign of brain death. CT can be normal in the early stages but generally becomes positive within 7–10 days in an area of infarction. In hemorrhage or hemorrhagic infarction, CT is excellent to demonstrate the presence of blood. Prior to in vivo measurements of glucose metabolism, CBF, and oxygen use with PET and energy metabolism by ^{1}H- and ^{31}P-NMR, electroencephalography (EEG) and evoked responses were the only methods available to follow brain function during life. In order to perform experimental metabolic studies, it was necessary to use intracarotid injections of isotopic tracers and to insert catheters into the jugular bulb for collection of samples to calculate arteriovenous differences. Recent technical advances now provide information on brain metabolism under in vivo conditions and open the way for the testing of new treatments.

With an increasing awareness of the underlying pathophysiological changes that take place in ischemic tissue, a number of promising treatments have become available. These include agents that reestablish the cerebral circulation, such as the fibrinolytic agent, tissue plasminogen activator, which dissolves blood clots, calcium channel blockers, which limit the entry of calcium into the cell and prevent the cascade of cell damage triggered by calcium, and glutamate receptor antagonists, which prevent amino acid activation of ionic influx. These and other agents act to enhance recovery. The mechanism of action of some potential pharmacological agents, such as amphetamines, opioid, neuropeptide antagonists, and gangliosides, is under investigation. These classes of drugs have undergone preliminary testing, and there are others that are still highly experimental.

8.2 HYPOXIA–ISCHEMIA IN CARDIAC ARREST

Cardiac arrest produces both anoxia and ischemia. Within 7–12 seconds of a heart arrest, there is loss of consciousness. There is systemic acidosis due to the anaerobic conditions and the build-up of lactate. Hypoxia and acidosis lead to changes in vascular tone, with dilatation and an increase in blood volume. Biochemical changes in the blood are more severe during a prolonged arrest and lead to a greater degree of brain damage. When the cardiac arrest occurs out of the hospital, there is a worse prognosis than if it occurs within the hospital. If cardiopulmonary resuscitation is performed very early after the arrest and circulation to the brain can be restored effectively, the extent of brain damage can be limited. Often, however, the lag between the arrest and the restoration of function is too long to permit a return of normal brain function. In a series of 459 patients who had an out-of-hospital cardiac arrest, 39 percent of those examined never regained consciousness, and of the 280 patients who awakened, 91 had persistent neurologic deficits (Longstreth et al., 1983).

The type of neurological damage that occurs secondary to a cardiac arrest is variable. In some patients, particularly younger patients, there is a period of confusion on regaining consciousness that clears with time. Generally, however, there is at least a decline in memory, probably related to the damage to the hippocampal cells. This can be mild and not interfere with normal function, or it can be an incapacitating amnesia. Some patients who survive are left with a global impairment in intellectual function. These patients are demented, but the dementia does not progress as occurs with degenerative processes, such as Alzheimer's disease. When the hypoxic–ischemic insult is severe, the patient who survives often remains comatose with the eyes open and with preservation of some primitive functions. This has been termed the "persistent vegetative state" (Jennett and Plum, 1972). Such patients are unaware of their surroundings but, with primitive functions preserved, appear to be awake. Thus, the severity of brain damage in patients surviving cardiopulmonary resuscitation can range from mild memory loss to severe dementia or persistent vegetative state (Willoughby and Leach, 1974; Snyder et al., 1977; Earnest et al., 1979).

A large, multicentered study determined the factors affecting recovery in a group of patients with nontraumatic or drug-induced comas (Levy et al., 1981). The majority of the patients had hypoxia–ischemia caused by cardiac arrest. As would be expected, those individuals who were awake soon after the arrest had the best prognosis for full recovery, whereas those showing a loss of brainstem function had the worst prognosis. Of the 120 patients with absent pupillary or corneal responses, only 1 regained function. The patients were in coma with their eyes closed for about 1 week before they evolved into the persistent vegetative state in which their eyes were open but there was no evidence of awareness or comprehension. Recovery from a vegetative state is rare. Younger patients with head injury or drug overdose may recover, and in extremely rare circumstances, an adult with a hypoxic–ischemic insult will regain some function (Rosenberg, et al. 1977). In the group of patients who fall between those who are awake shortly after the onset of coma and those who become vegetative, prediction of recovery is difficult. PET studies of CBF and glucose metabolic rate separated a group of patients who were in a persistent vegetative state from those who were locked-in because of brainstem infarcts that left them awake but totally paralyzed (Levy et al., 1987). The glucose metabolic rate was reduced to 50–60 percent of normal in the patients in the persistent vegetative state. Depression of metabolism was seen in all regions measured (Figure 8–1). Locked-in patients had preserved metabolic function.

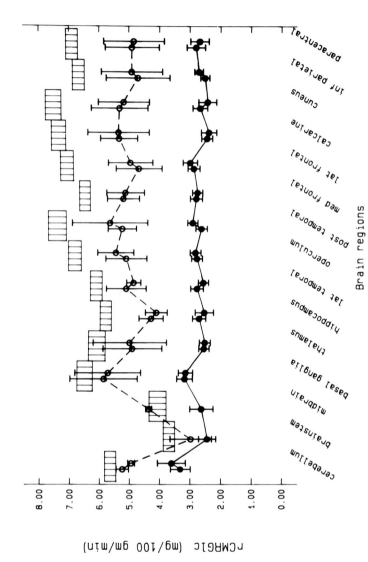

Figure 8–1. Cerebral metabolic rate for glucose (rCMRGlc) in different brain regions of normal, vegetative, and locked-in patients. For all regions except the brainstem and midbrain, the symbol to the left represents the left-sided structure and that to the right, the right-sided structure. The hatched boxes are mean ± SEM for 18 normal subjects. Circles and error bars are the mean ± SEM; solid circles represent 7 vegetative patients, and open circles represent 3 locked-in patients. lat, lateral; post, posterior; med, medial; inf, inferior. (From Levy et al., 1987)

The chances of regaining independent function after nontraumatic coma are shown in Table 8–1. Patients with metabolic causes of coma had the best chance of regaining function, and those with stroke had the worst prognosis. The patients with hypoxia–ischemia due to cardiac arrest had only a 12 percent chance of recovery.

Less severe episodes of hypoxia–ischemia can lead to milder cerebral damage. Patients undergoing cardiac surgery are at risk for subtle changes secondary to hypoxia–ischemia during the surgery (Sotaniemi, 1980). This is particularly true of elderly individuals with long hypotensive periods during surgery (Tufo et al., 1970). These patients frequently are confused on awakening from surgery, and an occasional patient is left with permanent amnesia or dementia.

In patients with anoxic damage after cardiac surgery, the type of surgery is related to the cerebral deficit (Furlan and Breuer, 1984). Replacement of damaged and infected heart valves results in a high incidence of embolic strokes. Coronary bypass surgery, particularly in its early days, was complicated occasionally by stroke but primarily by diffuse symptomatology, such as confusion and memory loss (Breuer et al., 1983). Patients were noted to be disoriented after surgery, which was originally attributed to a psychosis from the intensive care environment but, in retrospect, probably was due to abnormal metabolism.

Up to 80 percent of patients undergoing coronary artery bypass surgery show diffuse cerebral impairment in the immediate postoperative period, which has been suggested to be related to an initial hypocapnia at the onset of the operation and a subsequent hypercapnia (Nevin et al., 1987). The degree of transient neuropsychometric deficit was reduced in a group of patients in whom the P_{CO_2} was controlled more carefully. Although the majority of patients recovered without problems, one third still have deficits at 1 year postoperatively.

8.3 ANIMAL MODELS OF HYPOXIA–ISCHEMIA

Several animal models have been used to analyze brain hypoxic–ischemic damage (Table 8–2). Graded hypoxia is produced by substitution of nitrogen for oxygen. Hypoxia results from agents that poison oxidative metabolism or the oxygen-carrying capacity of hemoglobin. Cyanide injection produces

Table 8–1. Chances of Regaining Independent Function after Nontraumatic Coma in 500 Patients

Cause of Coma	Chance of Recovery (%)
Stroke	8
Hepatic encephalopathy	35
Other metabolic comas	34
Subarachnoid hemorrhage	13
Hypoxic–ischemic	12

From Levy et al., 1981.

Table 8–2. Experimental Models of Hypoxia–Ischemia

Type of Injury	Method of Induction
Hypoxia	
Hypoxic hypoxia	Substitution of O_2 with N_2
Chemical hypoxia	Cyanide poisoning
Hypoxia–Ischemia	Carotid ligation with O_2 deprivation
Ischemia	
Unilateral	Carotid occlusion in gerbil
Bilateral	Four-vessel occlusion
	Two-vessel occlusion with hypotension
Hemorrhagic	Direct injection of blood
	Ischemia with hypertension
	Postinfarction

anoxia by reacting with cytochrome oxidase and binding to hemoglobin. Carbon monoxide combines with hemoglobin to form carboxyhemoglobin, which is unable to carry oxygen. The toxicity of CO is due to the hypoxia resulting from its effect on hemoglobin, but CO also reacts with cytochrome oxidase and interferes with oxidation (Siesjo, 1978).

Brain ischemia is difficult to induce reproducibly in animals because of the collateral circulation from external to internal carotid and around the circle of Willis. Ischemia has been produced by several methods in rat, ranging from carotid occlusion with hypoxia (Levin, 1960) to cauterization of the vertebrals and occlusion of the carotids (Pulsinelli and Brierley, 1979). Regional ischemia has been produced by occlusion of the middle cerebral artery through the orbit (O'Brien and Waltz, 1973; Molinari et al., 1974). Global ischemia has been produced by inflation of a cuff around the neck or intrathoracic artery occlusion (Hossmann, 1982). A major problem with each of these models that limits their application is the variability from animal to animal, so that large numbers of animals often are needed.

Unilateral or bilateral carotid occlusion in the gerbil has been used as a model to study the time course in evolution of the ischemic lesion (Levine and Payan, 1966). Gerbils have an incomplete circle of Willis, so that unilateral carotid occlusion results in strokes on the ipsilateral side to the obstruction in approximately 40 percent of the animals. Seizures occur in some of the animals with stroke; this complicates interpretation of the data.

Models to simulate hemorrhage have been more difficult to produce. Hemorrhagic infarction was seen in animals with temporary occlusion of the middle cerebral artery and reperfusion (Hain et al., 1952; Crowell et al., 1970).

8.4 PATHOPHYSIOLOGY OF ANOXIA–ISCHEMIA

8.4.1 Hypoxia

There are many important similarities between the consequences of loss of oxygen and reduction in CBF. During hypoxia, oxygen falls, but there is normal or increased perfusion of the brain. Thus, oxidative metabolism comes to a halt while delivery of glucose to the brain continues. When blood flow to the brain falls below a critical threshold, delivery of both oxygen and essential nutrients is impaired. In ischemia, the energy substrates, such as PCr and ATP, decline, and degradative enzymes, such as lipases, that release free fatty acids are mobilized. Although there are differences in the events that lead to cell damage in both hypoxia and ischemia, the similarities in the two allow them to be discussed together.

The oxygen-carrying capacity of blood depends on multiple factors, including the level of hemoglobin, the temperature, the PCO_2, diphosphoglycerate, and the pH. Either raising the pH or lowering the temperature increases the oxygen saturation of blood, increasing oxygen uptake at the lung but decreasing oxygen release at the capillary. Hypoxia is accompanied by hyperventilation with hypocapnia and alkalosis.

Hypoxia can be induced in animals by substitution of nitrogen for oxygen. Reducing oxygen content of the inspired air from 30 percent to 10 percent lowers arterial oxygen from 90 mm Hg to 30 mm Hg. Table 8–3 shows the results of oxygen reduction on blood gases and cerebral function. Since higher altitudes have lower oxygen levels, the atmosphere at an altitude of 2,500 meters is equivalent to 15 percent oxygen, resulting in an alveolar PO_2 of around 70 mm Hg. Mild reductions in oxygen level are reported to impair the ability to learn a complex task (Ernsting, 1966). At 5,000 meters, the alveolar oxygen falls to around 40 mm Hg, and short-term memory can be affected (Crow and Kelman, 1971). Consciousness may be lost at an oxygen level of 30 mm Hg, which corresponds to over 8,000 meters above sea level.

Some measurements have been made at extreme altitudes during climbing expeditions at Mt. Everest (West, 1984). The cold and low oxygen result in a shift of the oxygen dissociation curve to the left, allowing greater oxygen-carrying capacity. Normally, at an atmospheric pressure of 760 mm Hg and 20 percent oxygen, the alveolar gas has a PO_2 of about 100 mm Hg, and there is a similar arterial blood gas. At high altitude, the barometric

Table 8–3. Effect of Acute Change in Oxygen on Cerebral Function

Altitude (meters)	Equivalent[a] FIO_2	PAO_2[b]	$PACO_2$ (mm Hg)	Clinical Impairment[c]
0	21	95	38	None
1,500	17	85	38	Dark adaptation
2,500	15	70	38	Concentration
3,000	14	60	36	Short-term memory
4,500	11	45	34	Critical judgment
6,000	9	35	30	Lethargy

[a]FIO_2 is the fractional equivalent of oxygen in inspired air in mm Hg.

[b]PAO_2 and $PACO_2$ are the alveolar pressures of oxygen and carbon dioxide, respectively.

[c]The clinical manifestations are variable and depend on multiple factors, including altitude and oxygen levels.

Modified from Gibson et al., 1981.

pressure is lower, and the inspired oxygen is reduced. Mountain climbers on Mt. Everest had an alveolar Po_2 of 35 mm Hg at 7,000 meters and a remarkable Pco_2 of 7.5 mm Hg with an arterial pH of 7.7 (West, 1984). Psychometric tests showed impairment of learning, memory, and expression of verbal material (West, 1986). Impairments in fingertapping speed persisted in climbers tested 12 months later. Persistent impairment in memory has been reported in mountain climbers who have climbed to extreme altitudes. Five of eight men who reached 8,000 meters without supplemental oxygen showed subtle defects in concentration, short-term memory, and ability to shift concepts (Regard et al., 1989).

Cerebral edema can occur in some individuals at high altitude. High altitude climbers have frequent headaches, but only a few have papilledema, lethargy, and coma. Fluid abnormalities may be involved because acetazolamide is able to block the effects of altitude sickness (Johnson and Rock, 1988). The influence of the level of Pco_2 in addition to the O_2 has been suspected for many years to be important in the evolution of pathological changes. Climbers with acute mountain sickness who are hypoxic with hypocapnia have been treated by raising the level of carbon dioxide in the inspired air. CBF has been measured under extremely difficult conditions in a small group of mountain climbers. By adding CO_2 to the inspired air, the CBF improved and the symptoms abated (Harvey et al., 1988).

The reason for the impairment of cerebral function at moderate levels of hypoxia is unclear. Attempts to relate energy state to cerebral function have shown that until the arterial oxygen levels fall below 20 mm Hg, there is preservation of ATP and PCr. A drop in oxygen to 13 percent produced an increase in lactate, and PCr fell at an oxygen level of 7 percent (Gurdjian et al., 1944). Levels of ATP are stable in rats made hypoxic until an oxygen content of 4 percent is reached (Gottesfeld and Miller, 1969). Lactate increased during hypoxia in rats anesthetized with nitrous oxide at an arterial oxygen of 40 mm Hg, whereas PCr fell at 30 mm Hg (Siesjo and Nilsson, 1971). Therefore, a loss of ATP and PCr explains the altered cerebral function that occurs with severe hypoxia but does not explain the impaired function with milder degrees of hypoxia.

Neurotransmitters are altered in hypoxia. Turnover of catecholamines and serotonin was found to be reduced in mild hypoxia (Davis et al., 1973). Oxygen levels of 50 mm Hg were sufficient to reduce the synthesis of acetylcholine (Gibson and Blass, 1976). Incorporation of ^{14}C-glucose and deuterated choline into acetylcholine was reduced with hypoxia, suggesting that reduced synthesis of neurotransmitters was the causative factor in cerebral impairment (Gibson et al., 1981).

Cerebral perfusion is preserved or increased in the early stages of hypoxia. However, as the compensatory hyperventilation lowers arterial Pco_2, there is vasoconstriction. The complex changes that occur during both hypoxia and hypocapnia have complicated the analysis. Furthermore, the heart is sensitive to hypoxia. In severe hypoxia, cardiac output falls, and hypotension augments the damage from hypoxia. The combination of hypoxia and hypotension is thus an additional factor to take into account when assessing the extent of permanent injury to cells.

8.4.2. Hypoxia–Ischemia

The combination of occlusion of a blood vessel with hypoxia in the rat leads to a hypoxic–ischemic injury. In mammals without collateral circulation between distant vascular territories, the distal tissue becomes ischemic when the carotid or the middle cerebral arteries are occluded. This is the situation in patients with stroke, in whom an occluded vessel in a poorly collateralized region produces an ischemic injury. Studies of ischemic injury have shown a multitude of changes that involve ions, amino acids, fatty acids, and so on. The complex nature of these changes and the number of them occurring over a short period of time make their analysis difficult. However, through studies focused on one or another of these changes, an overall picture of the progression in a damaged region has been obtained.

Hypoxia–ischemia produces complex biochemical changes. Initially, high-energy phosphates are depleted, and there is a shift of metabolism to anaerobic glycolysis. Normally, cellular function depends on ATPase for the pumping of sodium out of the cell and potassium into it across the plasma membrane. When levels of ATP fall, electrolytes are shifted from the extracellular space into the cell, and there is cell swelling. As potassium accumulates in the extracellular space, it interferes with neural transmission.

Although some cell types are more sensitive to damage and may be destroyed before others, eventually the membranes in neurons, glia, and blood vessels are damaged. A secondary event due to swelling in the endothelial cells is a reduction in CBF that interferes with blood flow when the circulation is restored so that there is no reflow of blood into the injured area (Ames et al., 1968). In experimental animals, recovery of electrical activity after prolonged cerebral ischemia has been observed (Hossmann and Sato, 1970).

8.4.3 Excitatory Neurotransmitters, Energy Charge, and Acidosis in Ischemia

Excitatory amino acids are toxic to neurons, and their neurotoxicity is proportional to their excitatory capacity (Rothman and Olney, 1986). Glutamate in excessive amounts leads to prolonged depolarization and synaptic activity with excessive sodium and calcium influx. In hippocampal slice preparations submitted to hypoxic conditions, glutamate produced prolonged depolarization, with ion and water influx from the extracellular space (Rothman, 1985). Cell damage from glutamate appears to occur in two phases: a rapid phase mediated by sodium and chloride influx with osmotic changes and a delayed phase related to the cellular events triggered by calcium influx (Figure 8–2). Excitatory amino acid neurotransmitters are decreased in ischemia in whole brain preparations, but their extracellular levels are increased in

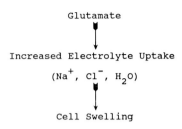

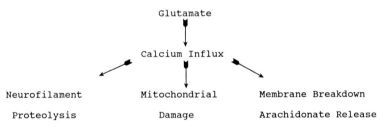

Figure 8–2. Ionic events involved in glutamate neurotoxicity. A. Rapid excitotoxic death probably is induced by an increased sodium permeability that results in depolarization, chloride entry, and eventually, osmotic lysis of swollen cells. B. Delayed neuronal death may be related to calcium entry, either through glutamate-activated channels or cation-sensitive channels. Some of the potentially damaging effects of elevated intracellular calcium levels are listed. (Modified from Rothman and Olney, 1986)

ischemia (Benveniste et al., 1984). The extracellular levels of the excitatory amino acids are related to cellular excitation.

Glutamate receptors on brain cells are classified by the type of compound that binds to them. Three types of glutamate receptors have been identified: kainate, quisqualate, and N-methyl-D-aspartate (NMDA). Although glutamate binds to all three types, the NMDA receptor has a greater affinity for aspartate. The glutamate receptors are densely located in the CA_1 zone of the rat hippocampus, an area selectively vulnerable to ischemia. Glutamate receptors are blocked in the presence of Mg^{2+} by several compounds that are structurally similar to glutamate (Nowak et al., 1984; Bradford, 1986). One of these receptor antagonists, 2-aminophosphonoheptanoic acid (APH), blocks ischemic changes in the rat hippocampus when it is injected directly into the structure (Simon et al., 1984b). Direct brain injection was needed because of the poor penetration of these agents across the blood–brain barrier.

Within seconds after the onset of ischemia, the levels of ATP and PCr begin to fall, reaching very low levels in 15 minutes. The fall in energy charge may be the trigger for the activation of phospholipases that begin the fatty acid release that leads to membrane damage. As intracellular calcium increases, the membrane phospholipases are activated. These, in turn, release free fatty acids. As membranes are damaged, there is no further influx of calcium (Farber et al., 1981).

With the onset of brain ischemia, potassium concentration increases in the extracellular space, stimulating its uptake into cells along with chloride in exchange for sodium and bicarbonate (Figure 8–3). The increase in intracellular ions causes astrocytes to swell, increasing the effects of ischemia. There is a compensatory increase in the metabolism of glucose and oxygen. Calcium and sodium concentrations in the extracellular fluid fall while intracellular concentrations increase. The damage is perpetuated further as intracellular calcium is increased when free fatty acids and sodium stimulate calcium release from endoplasmic reticulum and mitochondria. Normally, calcium is sequestered by the endoplasmic reticulum and accumulates in mitochondria by exchange with hydrogen.

The glucose blood level affects the extent of cellular damage. Fed animals had greater ischemic damage than starved animals, which was related to lactate build-up and acidosis (Myers 1979). Hyperglycemic animals were less likely to recover energy charge after hypoxia–ischemia than fasted animals, although there were no differences in the initial change in energy charge between the two groups. Brain pH measured by ^{31}P-NMR has shown a fall to 5.2 in markedly hyperglycemic animals (Chopp et al., 1987). This level is sufficiently low to lead to the activation of the lysosomal enzymes. Hyperglycemic animals show a marked increase in lactate, which is nor-

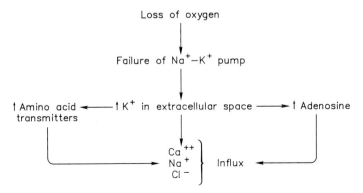

Figure 8–3. Sequence of changes in electrolytes and neurotransmitters initiated by hypoxia–ischemia.

mally less than 1 mM but can go as high as 40 mM. Lactate formation reduces NADH, which in turn forms ATP. As ATP is hydrolyzed, a proton is released. Normally, protons are buffered in the cell or removed in exchange for sodium. Excessive build-up of lactate can overwhelm both mechanisms, causing the cellular pH to fall low enough to activate lysosomal enzymes and produce lipid hydrolysis (Siesjo et al., 1985).

Newborns are more resistant to hypoxia–ischemia than are adults. Glucose in newborns is low in brain, and infusion of glucose protects against ischemia. Lactate transport is increased in newborns (Cremer et al., 1976). Immature animals appear to be better able to remove lactate from brain and may benefit from the excess energy provided by glucose metabolism. Whether newborns have the potential to metabolize lactate as a source of energy or have less need for oxidative metabolism is not well understood.

There is acidosis from lactate, ATP hydrolysis, and fatty acids. Levels of lactic acid in the injured tissue vary independently of the pH (Paschen et al., 1987). In complete ischemia, the correlation between the tissue lactic acid and pH was good, but in incomplete ischemia and in brain tumors, there was little correlation. They suggested that under anaerobic conditions the main source of proton production is ATP hydrolysis rather than glycolysis and that acidosis other than lactic acidosis appeared to be the damaging factor.

During hypoxia and ischemia, the neurotransmitter amino acids undergo complex changes. Synthesis of GABA by glutamic acid decarboxylase (GAD) continues, and its degradation by GABA-T is reduced. GAD has a pH optimum below 7, and it is inhibited by glutamate and ATP, both of which fall in ischemia, favoring the formation of GABA. In addition, the degradation of GABA by GABA-T is reduced in hypoxia, since it is dependent on the availability of the TCA cycle intermediate alpha-ketoglutarate. Thus, GABA will increase in hypoxia–ischemia.

8.4.4 Fatty Acid Metabolism in Ischemia

Another important factor in cell damage is the increase in free fatty acids. Increased levels of free fatty acids are found in severe hypoxia when oxygen levels are lowered to less than 30 mm Hg (Gardiner et al., 1981). The fatty acid showing the greatest increase is arachidonic acid. Ischemia also produces changes in the free fatty acid levels in the brain (Bazan, 1970).

Arachidonic acid produces a series of inflammatory mediators called "eicosanoids" (Wolfe, 1982). In the presence of oxygen, there is formation of prostaglandins, thromboxanes, and leukotrienes. Prostaglandin metabolism to prostacyclin (PGI_2) is inhibited; PGI_2 promotes vasodilatation and prevents platelet aggregation. In ischemia, there is formation of thromboxane A_2, which promotes platelet aggregation and vasoconstriction.

Normally, fatty acids are bound to membranes in phospholipids. The second messenger phosphatidylinositol (PI) uses a phospholipase in the activation of membrane receptors. As calcium enters the cell during depolarization, other lipases can be activated. Phospholipase A_2 acts on the phospholipid at the second position in the glycerol molecule to hydrolyze the fatty acids. The complex changes that occur in lipid membranes during hypoxia–ischemia are an important contributing factor in cell death.

The sources of free fatty acids include phosphatidylcholine, phosphatidylethanolamine, phosphatidylserine, PI, and triglycerides. When gerbils are rendered ischemic by carotid occlusion, the ATP energy charge falls (Abe et al., 1987). Phospholipase C becomes active and removes inositol groups from the PI, forming diacylglycerol. With continued ischemia, there appears to be activation of diacylglycerol lipase and monoacylglycerol lipase that release arachidonic acid (20:4) and stearic acid (18:0) (Figure 8–4).

The release of arachidonic acid triggers a cascade of events that result in the formation of toxic lipid metabolites (Samuelsson et al., 1987). Cyclooxygenase forms prostaglandins and thromboxanes in the presence of oxygen. Lipoxygenases form another group of compounds, leukotrienes, which are mediators of inflammation (Figure 8–5). Leukotrienes have been demonstrated in the CNS and may be important mediators of inflammation. Cyclooxygenase inhibitors, such as indomethacin, have not been shown to be effective in treatment of ischemia. Attempts are underway to find an inhibitor of lipoxygenase that lacks toxicity to other organs.

8.5 PET IN HYPOXIA–ISCHEMIA

PET provides dynamic measurements of CBF, cerebral metabolic rate of oxygen (CMRO₂), oxygen extraction (OEF), cerebral blood volume (CBV), and cerebral metabolic rate of glucose (CMRGlc) (Phelps et al., 1982). Shortly

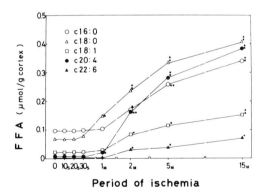

Period of ischemia

Figure 8–4. Changes in the content of free fatty acids (FFAs) during ischemia in gerbil cerebral frontoparietal cortexes. Periods of ischemia were 0 (sham control), 10 seconds, 20 seconds, 30 seconds, 1 minute, 2 minutes, 5 minutes, and 15 minutes, $n = 5$. SDs are within 15 percent of the mean values. Amounts of palmitic acid, stearic acid, arachidonic acid, and docosahexaenoic acid significantly increased during 15 minutes of ischemia ($p < 0.005$, $p < 0.001$). (From Abe et al., 1987)

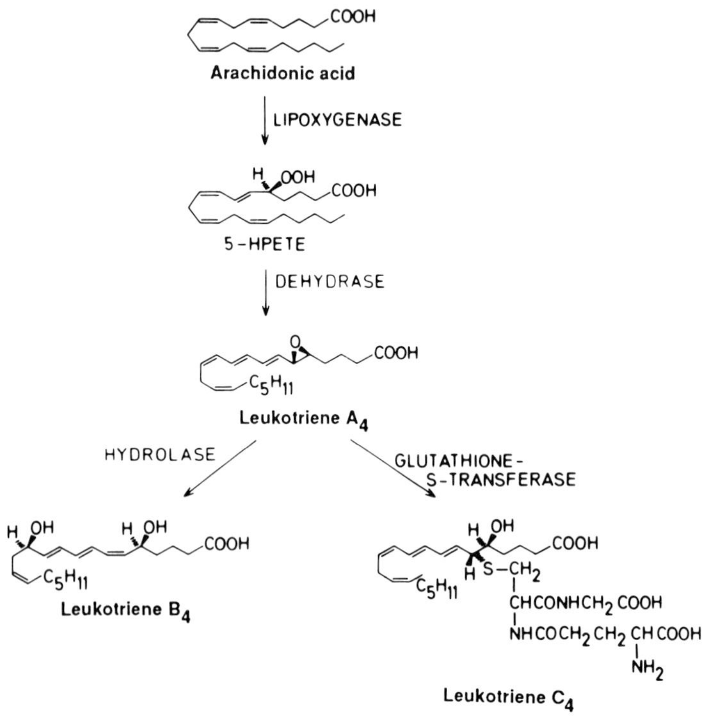

Figure 8–5. Oxygenation reactions involving arachidonic acid. (From Samuelsson et al., 1987)

after a fall in cerebral perfusion, there is vasodilatation, producing a compensatory increase in CBV. The OEF and $CMRO_2$ remain normal (Wise et al., 1983). With further decreases in perfusion pressure, the fall in oxygen delivery results in an increase in OEF, whereas $CMRO_2$ remains normal. At this preinfarction stage, the CBF is variable, and there is reduced OEF. As the damage progresses, there is a reduction in CBF, $CMRO_2$, and OEF.

After an infarct is established, the $CMRO_2$ can be decreased, as is the OEF, and the CBF is elevated. This elevation of CBF above metabolic demands is termed "luxury perfusion" and can be seen in strokes. PET studies have shown that CBF is an unreliable indicator of recovery. A better predictor appears to be the $CMRO_2$.

Occlusion of the internal carotid artery may lead to an increase in CBV in the ipsilateral hemisphere (Frackowiak, 1986). The increase in CBV means that resistance is lower and CBF is maintained in spite of the occlusion. A more advanced stage of injury is seen in some patients with maximally dilated vasculature ipsilateral to the carotid occlusion and a reduced CBF with an exhausted hemodynamic reserve.

Loss of tissue viability occurs in infarction. The ischemia preceding infarction shows a maximal rise in the OEF that is due to an attempt by the damaged tissue to remove as much oxygen as possible (Wise et al., 1983).

As the tissue infarcts, it lowers its metabolic rate. The reduced $CMRO_2$ remains low in spite of increased CBF, and the tissue changes generally are irreversible.

PET has shown the interplay of homeostatic mechanisms in ischemic tissue that lead to infarction. First, the cerebral vessels dilate to reduce peripheral resistance and maintain flow. When the hemodynamic reserve is exhausted and vasodilatation is maximal, the oxygen-carrying reserve increases. Finally, loss of both blood flow and oxygen extraction reserves leads to tissue infarction as the energy demands can no longer be met.

8.6 NMR IN HYPOXIA–ISCHEMIA

The ability of NMR to observe brain metabolism of ^{31}P in vivo was first shown to be feasible clinically in the study of hypoxic brain damage in infants (Cady et al., 1983). High-field strength magnets (1.9 T) of 30 cm bore were used to record ^{31}P spectra from the cerebral hemispheres of infants with birth anoxia due to various causes. Since the infants were critically ill, a nonmetallic transport incubator was constructed to avoid interference with the measurements. Both ^{31}P (32.5 MHz) and ^{1}H (80.3 MHz) resonance frequencies were used. The hydrogen molecule was used to show the location from the large water signal. A volume of tissue approximately 30 cm^3 was studied with a surface coil over a 10 minute collection period. Intracellular pH was measured from the difference in chemical shift between PCr and P_i. Since exact measurements of metabolites in a volume of tissue could not be done, the ratio of PCr/P_i was used. A normal infant had a ratio of 1.7, whereas infants with birth hypoxia–ischemia had ratios of less than 1. The lower ratio indicated a fall in the energy substrate, PCr, and an increase in P_i. In one infant, as the clinical state improved and after intravenous mannitol infusion, the ratio increased. There were no changes in pH in the anoxic infants.

Magnetic resonance spectroscopic measurements in animals with ischemia have been made on rabbits, rats, and gerbils. ^{31}P compounds have been measured in the brains of gerbils after 1 hour of carotid ligation (Thulborn et al., 1982). Simultaneous measurements were made of the brain water content, and no changes in brain water were seen until ^{31}P spectra were changed. In independent studies of the relationship of CBF to edema, it was demonstrated that edema occurred when blood flow fell to between 4 and 19 ml/g/minute. This implies that blood flow must be quite low before changes in the ^{31}P spectrum of ATP are observed.

With the design of high-field large-bore magnets, studies of adults with ischemia have become feasible. Using a 1.9 T meter bore magnet, patients with strokes have been studied (Bottomley et al., 1986). In stroke patients there is an initial acidosis that is related to the severity of the stroke, and the level of serum glucose, with a reversal to alkalosis when recovery occurs, and finally a return to normal pH (Figure 8–6) (Levine et al., 1988).

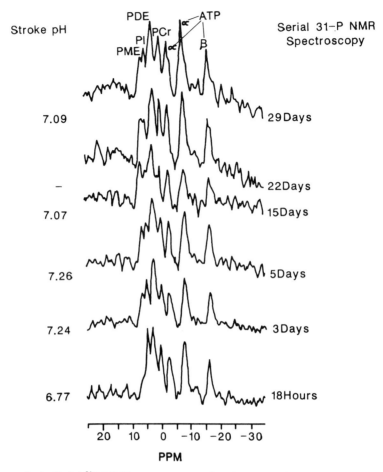

Figure 8–6. Serial ^{31}P-NMR spectroscopy of patient taken from the ischemic focus (CI). The inorganic phosphate (P$_i$) is elevated compared to the phosphocreatine (PCr) peak acutely, with gradual return to near normal ratio by 25 days. The CI pH is acidotic acutely, alkalotic subacutely, and returns to essentially normal levels by the later stages of the infarct evaluation. PME, phosphomonoesters; PDE, phosphodiesters. (From Welch et al., 1990)

^{31}P-NMR has been used to study hypoxia induced by cyanide poisoning in mice (Peres et al., 1988). Cyanide produced a fall in PCr and a rise in P$_i$ as seen with oxygen deprivation. However, the ATP levels were maintained by PCr metabolism to ATP, and the pH was only mildly reduced at a time when the electrical activity was lost. The delay in tissue acidosis was explained by either the consumption of protons by ATP synthesis from PCr or proton removal by the Na$^+$-H$^+$ antiporter. In another study of the effects of cerebral trauma on brain energetics, ^{31}P-NMR was used to monitor changes over several hours (Unterberg et al., 1988). Induction of injury in the cat by fluid–percussion of the cortex resulted in a fall of intracerebral pH for

30 minutes, with a return to baseline. No change was observed, however, in the PCr/P_i ratio or in the levels of ATP. Because of the mild nature of the changes, the fluid–percussion model was thought to not sufficiently mimic the conditions in a head-injured patient. Trauma to the spinal cord has been followed experimentally in rabbits with ^{31}P-NMR (Vink et al., 1987). Using a specially designed surface coil, they observed a fall in the PCr/P_i ratio and in the pH. By 4 hours after injury, the ratio fell from 2.7 to 0.5, while the pH dropped from 7.18 to 6.38.

^1H-NMR has been used either alone or in combination with ^{31}P-NMR to follow metabolic changes. Petroff et al. (1984) used combined ^{31}P-NMR and ^1H-NMR to study bicuculline-induced seizures. Lactate was shown to be elevated longer than the duration of the seizure. The signal attributed to lactate persisted in spite of a return of pH to normal. These studies were done using the lactate/N-acetylaspartate ratio, which may be affected by the membrane lipid signal near the lactate signal (Vink et al., 1988). In vivo measurements of hypoxia and ischemia differ from those in vitro, indicating problems with the use of ratios (Chang et al., 1987).

Lactate and pH measurements have been made in traumatic brain injury (McIntosh et al., 1987). During brain injury, there was a transient fall of brain pH along with a transient rise in the lactate level. The increase in lactate correlated with the fall in pH. However, the NMR changes were similar in moderately and severely injured animals, whereas functional recovery was worse in the severely injured animals. This suggests that factors other than lactate and pH are important for persistent deficits.

The effects of graded hypoxia have been studied in the rat using ^1H-NMR. A normoxic spectrum from a rat in a 7 T 89 mm bore magnet is shown in Figure 8–7. There is a large signal from the N-acetyl groups at 2.0 ppm, and other peaks are seen from the amino acids, primarily from glutamate at 2.3 ppm. With hypoxia, the signal at 2.0 ppm decreases and that from lactate at 1.3 ppm is seen to increase. After death, the lactate is markedly increased. The peaks have been identified in brain extracts (see Chapter 6).

8.7 THERAPEUTIC AGENTS IN ISCHEMIA

Therapy in stroke has taken several directions: (1) prevention of stroke by endarterectomy and anticoagulation, (2) reduction of edema by hyperosmolar agents, (3) improvement in blood flow with hemodilution, (4) blockade of calcium uptake by calcium entry blockers, and (5) prevention of neurotransmitter overstimulation by glutamate receptor antagonists.

Stroke prevention has been shown to be effective with control of hypertension and with antiplatelet aggregation agents. The role of carotid endarterectomy in stroke prevention is debated. It is probably an operation that is performed too frequently, and multicenter studies are underway to determine under which circumstances it is useful. Other forms of vascular surgery, such as temporal artery to middle cerebral artery bypass, have been

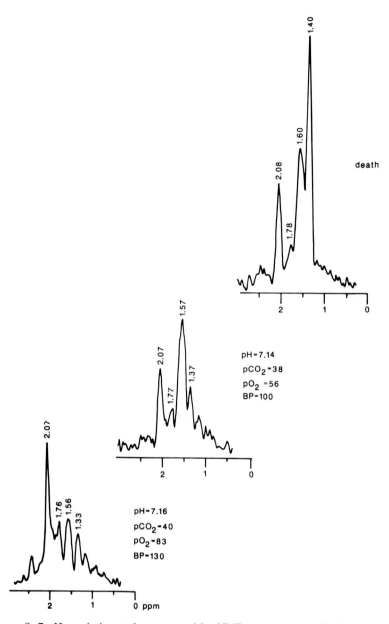

Figure 8–7. Hypoxia in rat demonstrated by NMR spectrometry. Surface coil and depth pulse were used. Bottom. ^{1}H-NMR of hypoxia in rat using surface coils. Lower left of figure shows characteristic peaks at 2.0 ppm from N-acetyl groups, 1.5–1.7 ppm from lipids, and 1.33 ppm from lactate. Middle. With reduction of oxygen, the 1.57 ppm signal increased. Top. When the animal died, a large rise in lactate occurred. (From Rosenberg et al., 1990)

shown to be of little use in stroke treatment (EC/IC Bypass Study Group, 1985).

Carotid endarterectomy is a very frequently performed surgical procedure. Indications for its use and complication rates vary from center to center. A consensus about its role in the treatment of transient ischemic attacks (TIAs) is lacking (Dyken, 1986). Patients with TIAs that are thought to be caused by emboli from the ipsilateral arteriosclerotic carotid artery generally are considered the best surgical candidates (Sandok et al., 1978). Aspirin and other antiplatelet agents have been shown to effectively lower the likelihood of stroke in patients with TIAs. However, the role of coumadin and heparin in the control of ischemic attacks is controversial.

Agents that dissolve formed blood clots have been used experimentally to reestablish flow in clotted coronary and carotid arteries. In an experimental model of embolic stroke, the infusion of tissue plasminogen activator reduced ischemic injury to the brain (Zivin et al., 1985). Clot lysis without induction of hemorrhage has been performed successfully with the clot-specific thrombolytic enzyme, tissue-type plasminogen activator. In an earlier series with another agent that lyses clots, streptokinase, there was an increase in mortality in drug-treated versus placebo-treated patients (Meyer et al., 1963). The danger of converting a nonhemorrhagic infarct into a hemorrhagic one is present with thrombolytic agents. The sooner the agents are given, the less the danger, but the therapeutic window, which is less than 4 to 6 hours, may be too short to be practical in many patients with stroke. Patients with myocardial infarction have been given tissue plasminogen activator with good success. A few of these patients have developed intracranial bleeding, but their number is small (2 of 386 patients in one series) (Califf et al., 1988). Myocardial infarction leads to cerebral infarction in a small number of patients, and those with hemorrhage after treatment with tissue plasminogen activator may have been in that group. However, stroke often leads to damage to the blood–brain barrier, so that treatment with tissue plasminogen activator after stroke may have a higher complication rate, as was found earlier with streptokinase.

After an acute stroke with brain swelling, the hyperosmolar agents, glycerol and mannitol, appear to improve recovery. These agents act by reducing water in normal tissue, since the blood–brain barrier damage in the infarcted region prevents an osmotic gradient. Patients previously were given 2–3 g/kg doses, but it is now known that 0.5–1 g/kg, which can be repeated at 4–6 hour intervals for several days, also is effective. The hyperosmotic agents selectively reduce water in the white matter and reduce the flow of interstitial fluid, which may be a factor in their therapeutic actions (Rosenberg et al., 1988). Use of steroids has not been found to be helpful in brain infarcts, and their use should be avoided.

Calcium channel entry blockers are a promising group of agents that have been used to reduce edema and the extent of injury in brain ischemia and hypoxia. Their use is based on the fact that calcium entry into cells is a major factor in the production of neuronal damage. The mechanism of action of the calcium antagonists is based on their ability to prevent influx of calcium into cells. Two mechanisms account for calcium entry, a voltage-sensitive and a receptor-sensitive mechanism. Normally, the extracellular fluid has millimolar concentrations of calcium, whereas the free intracellular calcium is 10,000 times less abundant (Greenberg, 1987). Voltage-sensitive channels are opened by membrane depolarization, and receptor-operated calcium channels are opened by neurotransmitters (Figure 8–8). Magnesium blocks the receptor-operated calcium channel and prevents calcium from entering the cell.

The major types of calcium channel blockers are shown in Table 8–4. The use of calcium channel antagonists has shown promising results in the treatment of stroke. Calcium antagonists, PN 200-110 and nimodipine, have been studied in a model of stroke in which the middle cerebral artery was occluded in stroke-prone, spontaneously hypertensive rats (Sauter and Rudin, 1986). Lesion evolution was followed by MRI at 24, 48, and 72 hours. Pretreatment or posttreatment with both antagonists significantly improved the infarct size and the neurobehavioral performance. In a subsequent study, they showed that the experimental calcium antagonists PY 108-068 and PN 200-110 both slowed the loss of high-energy phosphates as monitored by ^{31}P-NMR in a rat model of global ischemia (Sauter and Rudin, 1987). Al-

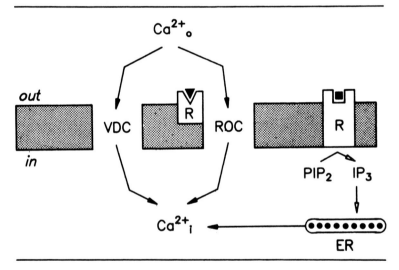

Figure 8–8. Cellular mechanisms for stimulus-evoked elevation of free intracellular calcium (Ca_i^{2+}). Extracellular calcium (Ca_o^{2+}) enters through voltage-dependent channels (VDC) opened by membrane depolarization or through receptor-operated channels (ROC) activated by the occupation of neurotransmitter receptors (R). Occupation of other receptors activates a phosphodiesterase that catalyzes the conversion of phosphotidylinositol 4,5-biphosphate (PIP_3) to inositol 1,4,5-triphosphate (IP_3). IP_3 acts on the endoplasmic reticulum (ER) membrane to release stored Ca^{2+} (filled circles) into the cytoplasm. (From Greenberg, 1987)

Table 8–4. Major Classes of Calcium Entry Blockers

Class	Drug
Dihydropyridines	Nifedipine (Procardia)
Phenylalkylamines	Verapamil (Calan)
Benzothiazepines	Diltiazem (Cardizem)
Diphenylalkylamines	Flunarizine

though the effect reached statistical significance, it was small, and the clinical relevance remains to be determined. The potential for these agents to produce hypotension and the need to give them before or shortly after the onset of the infarct may limit their clinical efficacy.

Several studies have shown that the antagonist, flunarizine, effectively reduces infarct size in a group of rats given the drug orally 3 hours before the insult (Van Reempts et al., 1987). The mechanism of flunarizine action may be to delay the calcium influx in neuronal and astrocytic cells. Flunarizine readily penetrates the blood–brain barrier, where it would have access to brain cells. The drug has multiple other actions on endothelial cells, platelets, and red blood cells. Which action is responsible for the protective effect remains to be determined.

Clinical trial of nimodipine in acute ischemic stroke showed a beneficial effect of early treatment in men (Gelmers et al., 1988). A prospective, placebo-controlled trial of nimodipine (30 mg every 6 hours) was carried out in 186 patients. Treatment was begun within 24 hours of the acute ischemic stroke. Fewer deaths occurred in the patients given nimodipine than with placebo; men were selectively helped by the drug. Although many questions remain to be answered, initial positive results have led to the clinical testing of other calcium channel blockers.

8.8 HYPOGLYCEMIA

Hypoglycemia is a life-threatening situation that occurs in insulin overdose, chronic alcoholism, neonates, Reye's syndrome, and rare inherited metabolic diseases, such as maple syrup urine disease. When glucose is low, amino acids and lipids become major substrates. Hypoglycemia is tolerated for longer periods than oxygen lack because of glucose, amino acids, and glycogen stores in the CNS, but persistent hypoglycemia leads to severe brain damage, with seizures and coma.

Overdoses of insulin from insulin-secreting tumors, self-injection of the drug, or iatrogenic causes result in hypoglycemia. Implantable devices to release insulin slowly have improved control of blood glucose levels. Closer control of serum glucose levels, however, increases the risk of hypoglycemic episodes. Unrecognized episodes of hypoglycemia have been documented during the night in insulin-dependent diabetics. Their occurrences can be masked by an early morning glucose increase. Occasionally, there is factitious hypoglycemia due to surreptitious insulin injections.

Glucose enters brain by carrier-mediated transport that can be modeled using formulas for enzyme kinetics. When glucose concentration in human plasma is 100 mg/dl (5.5 mM), the transport kinetic constants K_m and V_{max} in human brain are 6 μmol/g and 1.8 μmol/g/minute, respectively. Using as a normal intracellular glucose 3 mM, the resulting transport V_{net} is 0.3 μmol/g/minute. When plasma glucose falls to 3 mM and intracellular glucose is reduced to 1.25 mM, V_{net} remains unchanged. However, further decrease in plasma glucose leads to depletion of intracellular stores (Siesjo, 1978).

Oxygen consumption occurs at a rate of 1.6 μmol/g/minute and is exactly balanced by CO_2 production as expected if glucose is consumed as the main substrate (Sokoloff, 1989). Actually, the rate of glucose utilization is 0.3 μmol/g/minute, which is slightly higher than expected from oxygen consumption and indicates that glucose is incorporated into other substances and not completely consumed for energy use. In fact, a pool of substrates derived from glucose exists in the brain, so that the glucose being used at any given moment most likely was present in brain for some time, and newly acquired glucose has been incorporated in energy-storing molecules, such as glutamate, for later use.

Before the use of antipsychotic medications, insulin-induced hypoglycemia was used as a treatment in psychiatric disorders (Kety et al., 1948). In a study of hypoglycemia during insulin treatment in 14 schizophrenic patients, observations were made before intramuscular insulin injection, 90 minutes after injection, during coma, and after glucose infusion (Della Porta et al., 1964). The investigators found that CBF measured by the nitrous oxide method increased in coma, whereas the cerebral metabolic rate for glucose fell significantly, and the oxygen metabolic rate fell slightly. The respiratory quotient in comatose patients indicated the use of substrates other than carbohydrates. Thus, blood flow was increased, and oxygen metabolic rate was unchanged.

In animal studies of insulin hypoglycemia, it has been shown that the levels of ATP and PCr are maintained until blood sugar levels fall below 1 mM. Other metabolic changes include a reduction in NADH concentration, leading to a fall in the ratio of $NADH/NAD^+$ and persistent oxidation of redox systems, with a reduction of the malate/oxaloacetic acid ratio (Duffy and Plum, 1981).

Amino acids fall and ammonia levels rise in hypoglycemia. Glutamate combines with oxaloacetic acid to form aspartate and alpha-ketoglutarate. The fall in pyruvate leads to excess oxaloacetate, which leads to loss of glutamine, alanine, and GABA to provide additional glutamate (Norberg and Siesjo, 1976). Glutamate combines with NAD to form NADH and ammonia, and large amounts of ammonia accumulate. In addition, lipids are metabolized as an energy source. Membrane lipids are consumed when blood glucose levels fall below 20 mg/dl in rabbits (Hinzen et al., 1970).

8.9 HEPATIC ENCEPHALOPATHY

Liver failure occurs in a variety of pathological conditions, including alcoholic cirrhosis, infectious hepatitis, Reye's syndrome, Wilson's disease, and with certain toxins. Hepatic encephalopathy due to liver failure produces symptoms ranging from confusion to coma. Intermittent symptoms may be produced by ingestion of meals high in protein content in patients with hepatic insufficiency before complete liver failure. Characteristic pathological changes due to liver failure are seen in brain astrocytes, which have large, pale nuclei and prominent nucleoli (Norenberg, 1987). Elevated levels of ammonia are found and are thought to contribute to the metabolic disturbance in brain tissue. Improvement in cerebral symptoms follows correction of the high plasma ammonia either by treating the liver disease or by reducing ammonia formation in the gut with antibiotics, lactulose, and low-protein diet.

Elevated levels of ammonia may be the cause of the brain damage, but other possible toxins include short-chain fatty acids and false neurotransmitters. It is possible that a combination of several factors is involved. Ammonia labeled with positron-emitting ^{13}N has been used to show that its uptake and metabolism is a linear function of arterial concentration (Cooper and Plum, 1987). The response of the brain to ammonia varies with time of exposure. With prolonged exposure, the brain appears to have an increased sensitivity (Gjedde et al., 1978). Astrocytes are the primary cell involved in ammonia detoxification and show the greatest damage in hepatic encephalopathy. As the astrocytes degenerate, their ability to perform essential cellular functions is impaired. Astrocytes in cell culture exposed to ammonia show hypertrophic changes, followed by disturbances in membrane receptors and second messengers (Norenberg, 1987).

Ammonia is removed from the brain by several mechanisms. It is incorporated into glutamate from the TCA cycle intermediate, alpha-ketoglutarate. Glutamate forms glutamine in the presence of ATP, NH_4^+, Mg^{2+}, and phosphate by the action of glutamine synthetase. Patients with hepatic encephalopathy have increased levels of glutamine in CSF and blood, although glutamate levels are unchanged. Glutamic acid formation uses energy in the form of ATP and depletes the TCA cycle intermediates needed to reduce NAD^+ to NADH for subsequent use in the respiratory chain.

Glutamine formation takes place in the cytoplasm of astrocytes. Although the cause of cerebral disturbances in hepatic encephalopathy is debated, there is evidence that ammonia interferes with energy reserves, perhaps at the level of the malate–aspartate shuttle that normally transfers reducing equivalents from cytoplasm to mitochondria for oxidation (Hindfelt et al., 1977). One theory is that accumulation of ammonia in brain could inhibit malate–aspartate exchange by combining with cytoplasmic glutamate to form glutamine and thus deplete the mitochondria of substrate (NADH) for oxidative phosphorylation (Figure 8–9).

Another theory besides that of energy failure is that GABA levels are

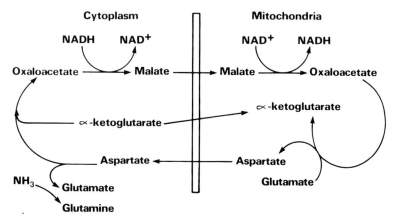

Figure 8–9. Transport of malate into mitrochondria may be important in generation of NADH needed to maintain respiration. Excess NH_3 would deplete glutamate. In the absence of glutamate, the formation of oxaloacetate would be decreased and the malate–aspartate exchange reduced. (Redrawn from Duffy and Plum, 1981)

elevated in serum and enter brain through an altered blood–brain barrier, where they inhibit normal neuronal function (Jones et al., 1984). Evidence for the GABA theory comes from the finding of elevated levels of GABA receptors in experimental animals (Baraldi and Zeneroli, 1982). GABA receptors are closely related to the benzodiazepine receptors, suggesting that these receptors, whose function in brain is unclear, may play a role in hepatic failure.

REFERENCES

Abe, K., Kogure, K., Yamamoto, H., Imazawa, M., Miyamoto, K.: Mechanism of arachidonic acid liberation during ischemia in gerbil cerebral cortex. J. Neurochem. 48:503–509, 1987.

Ames, A., III, Wright, R. L., Kowada, M., Thurston, J. M., Majno, G.: Cerebral ischemia. II. The no-reflow phenomenon. Am. J. Pathol. 52:437–453, 1968.

Baraldi, M., Zeneroli, Z. L.: Experimental hepatic encephalopathy: Changes in the binding of gamma-aminobutyric acid. Science 216:427–429, 1982.

Bazan, N. G., Jr.: Effects of ischemia and electroconvulsive shock on free fatty acid pool in the brain. Biochim. Biophys. Acta 218:1–10, 1970.

Benveniste, H., Drejer, J., Schousboe, A., Diemer, N. H.: Elevation of the extracellular concentrations of glutamate and aspartate in rat hippocampus during transient cerebral ischemia monitored by intracerebral microdialysis. J. Neurochem. 43:1369–1374, 1984.

Bradford, H. F.: Chemical Neurobiology: An Introduction of Neurochemistry. New York: W. H. Freeman and Co., 1986, pp. 219–225.

Breuer, A. C., Furlan, A. J., Hanson, M. R., Lederman, R. J., Loop, F. D., Cosgrove, D. M., Greenstreet, R. L., Estafanous, F. G.: Central nervous system complications of coronary artery bypass graft surgery: Prospective analysis of 421 patients. Stroke 14:682–687, 1983.

Cady, E. B., Costello, A. M., Dawson, M. J., Delpy, D. T., Hope, P. L., Reynolds, E. O., Tofts, P. S., Wilkie, D. R.: Non-invasive investigation of cerebral metabolism in newborn infants by phosphorus nuclear magnetic resonance spectroscopy. Lancet 1:1059–1062, 1983.

Califf, R. M., Topol, E. J., George, B. S., Boswick, J. M., Abbottsmith, C., Sigmon, K. N., Candela, R., Masek, R., Kereiakes, D., O'Neill, W. W., Stack, R. S., Stump, D.: Hemorrhagic complications associated with the use of intravenous tissue plasminogen activator in treatment of acute myocardial infarction. Am. J. Med. 85:353–359, 1988.

Chang, L. H., Pereira, B. M., Weinstein, P. R., Keniry, M. A., Murphy-Boesch, J., Litt, L., James, T. L.: Comparison of lactate concentration determinations in ischemic and hypoxic rat brains by in vivo and in vitro ^{1}H-NMR spectroscopy. Magnet. Reson. Med. 4:575–581, 1987.

Chopp, M., Glasberg, M. R., Riddle, J. M., Hetzel, F. W., Welch, K. M.: Photodynamic therapy of normal cerebral tissue in the cat: A noninvasive model for cerebrovascular thrombosis. Photochem. Photobiol. 46:103–108, 1987.

Cooper, A. J., Plum, F.: Biochemistry and physiology of brain ammonia. Physiol. Rev. 67:440–519, 1987.

Cremer, J. E., Braun, L. D., Oldendorf, W. H.: Changes during development in transport processes of the blood–brain barrier. Biochim. Biophys. Acta 448:633–637, 1976.

Crow, T. J., Kelman, G. R.: Effect of mild acute hypoxia on human short-term memory. Br. J. Anaesth. 43:548–552, 1971.

Crowell, R. M., Olsson, Y., Klatzo, I., Ommaya, A.: Temporary occlusion of the middle cerebral artery in the monkey. Clinical and pathological observations. Stroke 1:439–448, 1970.

Davis, J. N., Carlsson, A., MacMillan, V., Siesjo, B. K.: Brain tryptophan hydroxylation: Dependence on arterial oxygen tension. Science 182:72–74, 1973.

Della Porta, P. A., Maiolo, A. T., Negri, V. U., Rossella, E.: Cerebral blood flow and metabolism in therapeutic insulin coma. Metabolism 13:131–140, 1964.

Duffy, T. E., Plum, F.: Seizures, coma and major metabolic encephalopathies. In Basic Neurochemistry (Siegel, G. J., Albers, R. W., Agranoff, B. N., Katzman, R., eds.), Boston: Little, Brown and Company, 1981, pp. 693–718.

Dyken, M. L.: Carotid endarterectomy studies: A glimmering of science. Stroke 17:355–358, 1986.

Earnest, M. P., Breckinridge, J. C., Yarnell, P. R., Oliva, P. B.: Quality of survival after out-of-hospital cardiac arrest: Predictive value of early neurologic evaluation. Neurology 29:56–60, 1979.

EC/IC Bypass Study Group: Failure of extracranial–intracranial arterial bypass to reduce the risk of ischemic stroke. N. Engl. J. Med. 313:1191–1200, 1985.

Ernsting, J.: The effects of hypoxia upon human performance and the electroencephalogram. Int. Anesthesiol. Clin. 4:245–259, 1966.

Farber, J. L.: The role of calcium in cell death. Life Sci. 29:1289–1295, 1981.

Frackowiak, R. S.: PET scanning: Can it help resolve management issues in cerebral ischemic disease? Stroke 17:803–807, 1986.

Furlan, A. J., Breuer, A. C.: Central nervous system complications of open heart surgery. Stroke 15:912–915, 1984.

Gardiner, M., Nilsson, B., Rehncrona, S., Siesjo, B. K.: Free fatty acids in the rat brain in moderate and severe hypoxia. J. Neurochem. 36:1500–1505, 1981.

Gelmers, H. J., Gorter, K., de Weerdt, C. J., Wiezer, H. J. A.: A controlled trial of nimodipine in acute ischemic stroke. N. Engl. J. Med. 318:203–207, 1988.

Gibson, G. E., Blass, J. P.: Impaired synthesis of acetylcholine in brain accompanying mild hypoxia and hypoglycemia. J. Neurochem. 27:37–42, 1976.

Gibson, G. E., Pulsinelli, W., Blass, J. P., Duffy, T. E.: Brain dysfunction in mild to moderate hypoxia. Am. J. Med. 70:1247–1254, 1981.

Gjedde, A., Lockwood, A. H., Duffy, T. E., Plum, F.: Cerebral blood flow and metabolism in chronically hyperammonemic rats: Effect of an acute ammonia challenge. Ann. Neurol. 3:325–330, 1978.

Gottesfeld, Z., Miller, A. T., Jr.: Metabolic response of rat brain to acute hypoxia: Influence of polycythemia and hypercapnia. Am. J. Physiol. 216:1374–1379, 1969.

Greenberg, D. A.: Calcium channels and calcium channel antagonists. Ann. Neurol. 21:317–330, 1987.

Gurdjian, E. S., Stone, W. E., Webster, J. E.: Cerebral metabolism in hypoxia. Arch. Neurol. Psych. 54:472–477, 1944.

Hain, R. F., Westhayesen, P. U., Swank, R. L.: Hemorrhagic cerebral infarction by arterial occlusion. J. Neuropathol. Exp. Neurol. 11:34–43, 1952.

Harvey, T. C., Raichle, M. E., Winterborn, M. H., Jensen, J., Lassen, N. A., Richardson, N. V., Bradwell, A. R.: Effect of carbon dioxide in acute mountain sickness: A rediscovery. Lancet 2:639–641, 1988.

Hindfelt, B., Plum, F., Duffy, T. E.: Effect of acute ammonia intoxication on cerebral metabolism in rats with portacaval shunts. J. Clin. Invest. 59:386–396, 1977.

Hinzen, D. H., Becker, P., Muller, U.: Einfluss von Insulin auf den regionalen Phospholipidstoff wechsel des Kaninchengehirns in vivo. Pflugers Arch. 321:1–14, 1970.

Hossmann, K. A.: Treatment of experimental cerebral ischemia. J. Cereb. Blood Flow Metab. 2:275–297, 1982.

Hossmann, K. A., Sato, K.: Recovery of neuronal function after prolonged cerebral ischemia. Science 168:375–376, 1970.

Jennett, B., Plum, F.: Persistent vegetative state after brain damage: A syndrome in search of a name. Lancet 1:734–737, 1972.

Johnson, T. S., Rock, P. B.: Acute mountain sickness. N. Engl. J. Med. 319:841–845, 1988.

Jones, E. A., Schafer, D. F., Ferenci, P., Pappas, S. C.: The neurobiology of hepatic encephalopathy. Hepatology 4:1235–1242, 1984.

Kety, S. S., Woodford, R. B., Harmel, M. H., Freyhan, F. A., Appel, K. E., Schmidt, C. F.: Cerebral blood flow and metabolism in schizophrenia: The effects of barbiturate semi-narcosis, insulin coma and electroshock. Am. J. Psychiatry 104:765–770, 1948.

Levine, S.: Anoxic–ischemic encephalopathy in rats. Am. J. Pathol. 36:1–17, 1960.

Levine, S., Payan, H.: Effects of ischemia and other procedures on the brain and retina of the gerbil (Meriones unguiculatus). Exp. Neurol. 16:255–262, 1966.

Levine, S. R., Welch, K. M., Helpern, J. A., Chopp, M., Bruce, R., Selwa, J., Smith, M. B.: Prolonged deterioration of ischemic brain energy metabolism and acidosis associated with hyperglycemia: Human cerebral infarction studied by serial ^{31}P NMR spectroscopy. Ann. Neurol. 23:416–418, 1988.

Levy, D. E., Bates, D., Caronna, J. J., Cartlidge, N. E., Knill Jones, R. P., Lapinski, R. H., Singer, B. H., Shaw, D. A., Plum, F.: Prognosis in nontraumatic coma. Ann. Intern. Med. 94:293–301, 1981.

Levy, D. E., Sidtis, J. J., Rottenberg, D. A., Jorden, J. O., Strother, S. C., Dhawan, V., Ginos, J. Z., Tramo, M. J., Evans, A. C., Plum, F.: Differences in cerebral blood flow and glucose utilization in vegetative versus locked-in patients. Ann. Neurol. 22:673–682, 1987.

Longstreth, W. T., Jr., Inui, T. S., Cobb, L. A., Copass, M. K.: Neurologic recovery after out-of-hospital cardiac arrest. Ann. Intern. Med. 98:588–592, 1983.

McIntosh, T. K. Faden, A. I., Bendall, M. R., Vink, R.: Traumatic brain injury in the rat: Alterations in brain lactate and pH as characterized by ^{1}H and ^{31}P nuclear magnetic resonance. J. Neurochem. 49:1530–1540, 1987.

Meyer, J. S., Gilroy, J., Barahart, M. I., Johnson, J. F.: Therapeutic thrombolysis in cerebral thromboembolism. Double-blind evaluation of intravenous plasmin therapy in carotid and middle cerebral artery occlusion. Neurology 13:927–937, 1963.

Molinari, G. F., Moseley, J. I., Laurent, J. P.: Segmental middle cerebral artery occlusion in primates: An experimental method requiring minimal surgery and anesthesia. Stroke 5:334–339, 1974.

Myers, R. E.: A unitary theory of causation of anoxic and hypoxic brain pathology. Adv. Neurol. 26:195–213, 1979.

Nevin, M., Adams, S., Colchester, A. C. F., Pepper, J. R.: Evidence for involvement of hypocapnia and hypoperfusion in aetiology of neurological deficit after cardiopulmonary bypass. Lancet 2:1493–1495, 1987.

Norberg, K., Siesjo, B. K.: Oxidative metabolism of the cerebral cortex of the rat in insulin-induced hypoglycemia. J. Neurochem. 26:345–52, 1976.

Norenberg, M. D.: The role of astrocytes in hepatic encephalopathy. Neurochem. Pathol. 6:13–33, 1987.

Nowak, L., Bregestovski, P., Ascher, P., Herbet, A., Prochiantz, A.: Magnesium gates glutamate-activated channels in mouse central neurones. Nature 307:462–465, 1984.

O'Brien, M. D., Waltz, A. G.: Transorbital approach for occluding the middle cerebral artery without craniectomy. Stroke 4:201–206, 1973.

Paschen, W., Djuricic, B., Mies, G., Schmidt-Kastner, R., Linn, F.: Lactate and pH in the brain: Association and dissociation in different pathophysiological states. J. Neurochem. 48:154–159, 1987.

Peres, M., Meric, P., Barrerre, B., Pasquier, C., Beranger, G., Beloeil, J. C., Lallemand, J. Y., Seylaz, J.: In vivo ^{31}P nuclear magnetic resonance (NMR) study of cerebral metabolism during histotoxic hypoxia in mice. Metab. Brain Dis. 3:37–48, 1988.

Petroff, O. A., Prichard, J. W., Behar, K. L., Alger, J. R., Shulman, R. G.: In vivo phosphorus nuclear magnetic resonance spectroscopy in status epilepticus. Ann. Neurol. 16:169–177, 1984.

Phelps, M. E., Mazziotta, J. C. Huang, S. C.: Study of cerebral function with positron computed tomography. J. Cereb. Blood Flow Metab. 2:113–162, 1982.

Pulsinelli, W. A., Brierley, J. B.: A new model of bilateral hemispheric ischemia in the unanesthetized rat. Stroke 10:267–272, 1979.

Pulsinelli, W. A., Duffy, T. E.: Local cerebral glucose metabolism during controlled hypoxemia in rats. Science 204:626–629, 1979.

Regard, M., Oelz, D., Brugger, P., Landis, T.: Persistent cognitive impairment in climbers after repeated exposure to extreme altitude. Neurology 39:210–213, 1989.

Rosenberg, G. A., Johnson, S. F., Brenner, R. P.: Recovery of cognition after prolonged vegetative state. Ann. Neurol. 2:167–169, 1977.

Rosenberg, G. A., Barrett, J., Estrada, E., Brayer, J., Kyner, W. T.: Selective effect of mannitol-induced hyperosmolality on brain interstitial fluid and water content in white matter. Metab. Brain Dis. 3:217–227, 1988.

Rosenberg, G. A., Kyner, E., Gasparovic, C., Griffey, R. H., Matwiyoff, N. A.: ^{1}H-NMR spectroscopy in brain. In: *NMR: Principles and Applications to Biomedical Research* (Pettegrew, J. editor), New York: Springer-Verlag, 1990:468–484.

Rothman, D. L., Behar, K. L., Hetherington, H. P., den Hollander, J. A., Bendall, M. R., Petroff, O. A., Shulman, R. G.: ^{1}H-Observe/^{13}C-decouple spectroscopic measurements of lactate and glutamate in the rat brain in vivo. Proc. Natl. Acad. Sci. USA 82:1633–1637, 1985.

Rothman, D. L., Behar, K. L., Hetherington, H. P., Shulman, R. G.: Homonuclear ^{1}H double-resonance difference spectroscopy of the rat brain in vivo. Proc. Natl. Acad. Sci. USA 81:6330–6334, 1984.

Rothman, S. M.: The neurotoxicity of excitatory amino acids is produced by passive chloride influx. J. Neurosci. 4:1884–1891, 1985.

Rothman, S. M., Olney, J. W.: Glutamate and the pathophysiology of hypoxic–ichemic brain damage. Ann. Neurol. 19:105–111, 1986.

Samuelsson, B., Dahlen, S. E., Lindgren, J. A., Rouzer, C. A., Serhan, C. N.: Leukotrienes and lipoxins: Structures, biosynthesis, and biological effects. Science 237:1171–1176, 1987.

Sandok, B. A., Furlan, A. J., Whisnant, J. P., Sundt, T. M.: Guidelines for the management of transient ischemic attacks. Mayo Clin. Proc. 53:665–674, 1978.

Sauter, A., Rudin, M.: Calcium antagonists reduce the extent of infarction in rat middle cerebral artery occlusion model as determined by quantitative magnetic resonance imaging. Stroke 17:1228–1234, 1986.

Sauter, A., Rudin, M.: Effects of calcium antagonists on high-energy phosphates in ischemic rat brain measured by ^{31}P-NMR spectroscopy. Magnet. Reson. Med. 4:1–8, 1987.

Siesjo, B. K.: *Brain Energy Metabolism*. Chichester, England: John Wiley & Sons, 1978.

Siesjo, B. K., Bendek, G., Koide, T., Westerberg, E., Wieloch, T.: Influence of acidosis on lipid peroxidation in brain tissues in vitro. J. Cereb. Blood Flow Metab. 5:253–258, 1985.

Siesjo, B. K., Nilsson, L.: The influence of arterial hypoxemia upon labile phosphates and upon extracellular and intracellular lactate and pyruvate concentrations in the rat brain. Scand. J. Clin. Lab. Invest. 27:83–96, 1971.

Simon, R. P., Griffiths, T., Evans, M. C., Swan, J. H., Meldrum, B. S.: Calcium overload in selectively vulnerable neurons of the hippocampus during and after ischemia: An electron microscopy study in the rat. J. Cereb. Blood Flow Metab. 4:350–361, 1984a.

Simon, R. P., Swan, J. H., Griffiths, T., Meldrum, B. S.: Blockade of N-methyl-D-aspartate receptors may protect against ischemic damage in the brain. Science 226:850–852, 1984b.

Snyder, B. D., Ramirez Lassepas, M., Lippert, D. M.: Neurologic status and prognosis after cardiopulmonary arrest. I. A retrospective study. Neurology 27:807–811, 1977.

Sokoloff, L.: Circulation and energy metabolism of the brain. In *Basic Neurochemistry*. (Siegel, G. J., Agranoff, B. W., Albers, R. W., Molinoff, P. B., eds.) New York: Raven Press, 1989.

Sotaniemi, K. A.: Brain damage and neurological outcome after open-heart surgery. J. Neurol Neurosurg. Psychiatry 43:127–135, 1980.

Thulborn, K. R., du Boulay, G. H., Duchen, L. W., Radda, G.: A ^{31}P nuclear magnetic resonance in vivo study of cerebral ischemia in the gerbil. J. Cereb. Blood Flow Metab. 2:299–306, 1982.

Tufo, H. M., Ostfeld, A. M., Shekelle, R.: Central nervous system dysfunction following open-heart surgery. JAMA 212:1333–1340, 1970.

Unterberg, A. W., Andersen, B. J., Clarke, G. D., Marmarou, A.: Cerebral energy metabolism following fluid–percussion brain injury in cats. J. Neurosurg. 68:594–600, 1988.

Van Reempts, J., Van Deuren, B., Van de Ven, M., Cornelissen, F., Borgers, M.: Flunarizine reduces cerebral infarct size after photochemically induced thrombosis in spontaneously hypertensive rats. Stroke 18:1113–1110, 1987.

Vink, R., Knoblach, S. M., Faden, A. I.: ^{31}P magnetic resonance spectroscopy of traumatic spinal cord injury. Magnet. Reson. Med. 5:390–394, 1987.

Vink, R., McIntosh, T. K., Faden, A. I.: Nonedited ^{1}H-NMR lactate/N-acetyl aspartate ratios and the in vivo determination of lactate concentration in brain. Magnet. Reson. Med. 7:95–99, 1988.

Welch, K. M. A.: ^{31}P in vivo spectroscopy of adult human brain. In: *NMR: Principles and Applications to Biomedical Research* (Pettegrew, J., ed.) New York: Springer-Verlag, 1990, pp. 429–467.

West, J. B.: Hypoxic man: Lessons from extreme altitude. Aviat. Space Environ. Med. 55:1058–1062, 1984.

West, J. B.: Do climbs to extreme altitude cause brain damage? Lancet. 2:387–388, 1986.

Willoughby, J. O., Leach, B. G.: Relation of neurological findings after cardiac arrest to outcome. Br. Med. J. 3:437–439, 1974.

Wise, R. J. S., Bernardi, S., Frackowiak, R. S. J., Legg, N. J., Jones, T.: Serial observations on the pathophysiology of acute stroke: The transition from ischaemia to infarction as reflected in regional oxygen extraction. Brain 106:197–222, 1983.

Wolfe, L. S.: Eicosanoids: Prostaglandins, thromboxanes, leukotrienes, and other derivatives of carbon-20 unsaturated fatty acids. J. Neurochem. 38:1–14, 1982.

Zivin, J. A., Fisher, M., DeGirolami, V., Hemenway, C. C., Stashak, J. A.: Tissue plasminogen activator reduces neurological damage after cerebral embolism. Science 230:1289–1292, 1985.

9

Brain Edema

9.1 INTRODUCTION

Brain edema is a serious, often life-threatening occurrence that follows numerous insults to brain tissue. When edema develops, the prognosis for full recovery without damage to the nervous system is poor. Edema can occur after ischemia, trauma, tumors, and infections. Although the primary events may differ, the final biochemical disturbances are similar. If the edema can be prevented or reduced, chances of a normal recovery are greatly enhanced, and much research has been directed toward that goal.

Cerebral edema is defined as the accumulation of excess fluid either within cells or between them in the extracellular space (Klatzo, 1967) (Table 9–1). Cytotoxic edema is swelling of the cells. Vasogenic edema involves enlargement of the extracellular space with fluid from abnormally permeable blood vessels, and interstitial edema is the movement of CSF into the extracellular space of periventicular regions that are hydrocephalic (Fishman, 1975). Although edema may begin primarily as vasogenic or cytotoxic, as the process progresses, the injury leads to a combination of cellular swelling and vascular damage. Recent advances in imaging with CT and MRI have improved the diagnosis of brain edema. Attempts at treatment, however, have been less successful.

There is a complex relationship between increased CSF pressure and brain edema. Lumbar CSF pressure reflects the combined pressure from blood, CSF, and brain tissue. Since the skull of an adult is rigid, an increase in any one of the three compartments can result in an increase in the CSF pressure (Figure 9–1). For example, an increase in blood volume can increase intracranial pressure (ICP) without producing either cellular swelling or an increase in extracellular space. In other words, an increase in blood volume can increase ICP without producing brain edema. Conversely, brain

Table 9–1. Characteristics of Edema Types

Type	Pathology	Cause	Treatment
Vasogenic	Widened extracellular space in white matter; damaged blood–brain barrier	Brain tumors Trauma	Hyperosmolar agents Dexamethasone
Cytotoxic	Swollen cells with reduced extracellular space	Hypoxia Ischemia Toxins	Hyperosmolar agents
Interstitial	Transependymal and transpial fluid movement with widened extracellular space	Hydrocephalus	Ventriculoperitoneal shunt

tumors can cause edema or cellular and extracellular swelling, displacing blood and CSF without increasing CSF pressure. Understanding the causes of brain edema and increased ICP is important in planning the diagnostic approach to the patient.

The importance of differentiating various causes is seen in a condition called benign intracranial hypertension, or pseudotumor cerebri, in which there is an increase in CSF pressure with papilledema. In this condition, a lumbar puncture is safe and indicated to measure the pressure and remove fluid. However, when papilledema is due to a brain tumor, performing a lumbar puncture is not advised. Since the widespread use of CT and MRI, the dangers of inadvertently performing a lumbar puncture in the presence of a mass have been reduced greatly.

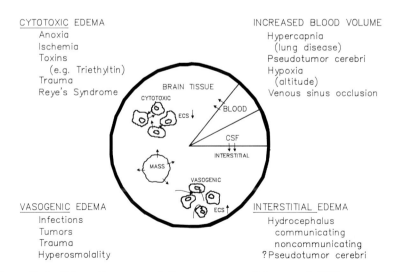

Figure 9–1. Schematic representation of causes of increased CSF pressure. Increased blood volume and CSF volume are shown on the right side. Cytotoxic edema reduces extracellular space (ECS), whereas vasogenic edema increases it. Masses result in vasogenic edema, and trauma produces both types.

9.2 INTRACRANIAL PRESSURE

Cerebrospinal fluid pressure in humans normally ranges from 80 to 180 mm H_2O. It is determined mainly by the pressure in the veins and sinuses draining blood from the head (Davson, 1967). Changes in arterial pressure are not reflected in CSF pressure except as fluctuations due to the cardiac pulse, since the muscular tension in the arterial wall counteracts the blood pressure.

The concept that the blood, CSF, and brain mass determine the ICP has been called the Monro-Kellie doctrine. Alexander Monro noted in 1783 that since the brain was incompressible and the skull rigid, the amount of blood leaving by the veins had to be the same as that entering by arteries. In 1824, George Kellie confirmed Monro's concept experimentally when he observed that animals killed by exsanguination had blood in the skull except where a trephine hole had been placed. George Burrows extended their observations in 1846 to include the CSF volume.

Since CSF pressure is closely related to venous pressure and, except in pathological situations, is independent of arterial pressure, the ICP increases when blood vessels dilate or venous outflow is impaired. For example, hypercapnia increases blood volume and CSF pressure (Ryder et al., 1953). Chronic hypoxia, as in patients with lung disease and in high altitude mountain climbers, causes vascular dilatation and can produce papilledema and headaches. Venous return to the heart is affected in lung diseases, such as emphysema, where papilledema is seen infrequently. The effects of hypoxia and hypercapnia are most pronounced in chronic lung disease with poor oxygenation of blood and carbon dioxide retention. The combination of hypoxia and hypocapnia produces a more variable effect on blood volume, which is difficult to predict.

The brain tissue compartment increases with cerebral masses, such as hemorrhage, tumors, or abscesses. Occasionally, a normal CSF pressure is found in patients with brain masses. Such masses may be accommodated by the brain because of their rate of growth or their location in a silent region of the brain. However, intracranial masses accompanied by edema are likely to cause papilledema.

As the CSF volume increases, there is a small compressive effect on the brain tissue. Blood is removed from the cerebral vessels, and the brain tissue itself is deformed. The amount of deformation secondary to compression is, however, limited. Initially, increases in CSF volume produce a small rise in pressure. Once the deformability of brain tissue is exceeded, more pronounced increases in pressure occur with each change in volume. Compliance is defined as the change in pressure with change in CSF volume. Compliance of brain tissue can be measured by injection of a small volume of fluid into the CSF space (Miller, 1975). As the pressure increases, smaller volumes of fluid produce greater increases in pressure, indicating less elasticity of the intracranial contents (Figure 9–2). Although of experimental interest, this has not been used as a clinical test.

Patients with suspected elevation of ICP can be monitored by insertion of

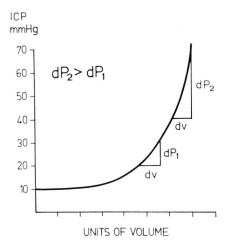

Figure 9–2. Theoretical intracranial volume–pressure curve. As volume increases and intracranial pressure (ICP) rises, uniform increments of volume (dV) cause larger and larger rises of intracranial pressure (dP). Intracranial elastance (dP/dV) thus increases in parallel with the intracranial pressure during progressive addition to the volume of the intracranial contents. (From Miller, 1975)

a catheter into the lateral ventricle for continuous pressure recording and assessment of results of treatment (Lundberg, 1960). In normal people and in patients with increased ICP, the intraventricular pressure fluctuates during the day. When the ICP is elevated, these fluctuations may produce periods of sustained pressure elevations, which have been called "B waves." The reason for these periods of very high pressure in patients with raised ICP is not understood. Frequently, they occur at night and may be due to hypoventilation. Although monitoring of ICP has been performed mainly in patients with head trauma or in children with Reye's syndrome, it has been used in other situations where the ICP is increased. The main complication is infection from the indwelling catheter, so that experienced nursing in an intensive care unit is necessary to reduce the incidence of infection and bleeding from the catheter site.

ICP monitoring has been used most extensively in head-injured patients. A poorer prognosis was found in patients with ICP elevated above 15 mm Hg. Very high pressure was associated with death (Marshall et al., 1979). The level of ICP elevation in head-injured patients reflects the extent of tissue injury and brain swelling. A poor outcome generally is related to the extent of the initial injury that secondarily leads to an increase in ICP. A further complicating factor in head-injured patients is the presence of a mass lesion that contributes to the increase in ICP and worsens the eventual outcome.

The ability to perfuse the brain depends on the difference between the ICP and the blood pressure. This difference is defined as the cerebral perfusion pressure. When the ICP is greater than the blood pressure, the cerebral perfusion pressure is reduced to zero, and no blood flows to the brain. The ischemia further compromises the cerebral metabolism. At this point, the possibility of recovering function is negligible; the patient is brain dead. In fact, absence of blood flow to the brain during cerebral angiography is used as a criterion for brain death and is required to make that diagnosis in some countries.

The optimal use of intracranial monitoring has not been established (Ropper, 1985). Patients with head injury have been most intensively monitored to optimize treatment with hyperosmolar agents. However, many centers do not routinely use pressure monitoring in the management of head-injured patients. Children with Reye's syndrome die from complications of brain edema and often are monitored with intracranial devices for assessment of treatment. Patients with brain tumors, stroke, increased blood volume, and metabolic coma rarely are followed with intracranial monitoring, since raised pressure generally is not the major cause of brain damage.

9.3 BRAIN EDEMA

9.3.1 Experimental Edema Models

Edema within brain cells and extracellular spaces produces secondary effects on brain metabolism and cerebral blood flow, increasing the extent of cellular damage. Analysis of the factors involved in cell damage has been aided by the use of experimental models of brain edema. Brain insults that have been used to cause edema are ischemia, hypotension, hypertension, trauma, and toxins (Table 9–2). Resistance of certain species and susceptibility of others to pathological changes is a complicating factor. For example, most animals have extensive collateral circulation through the circle of Willis and the extracranial vessels. Occlusion of a major blood vessel in the neck in these species has little effect. Therefore, production of hypoxia–ischemia requires either clamping of the aorta or unilateral carotid occlusion with hypoxia and hypoperfusion or occlusion of both anterior and posterior circulations (Pulsinelli et al., 1982). A further complicating factor is that extensive experimental manipulations make restoration of normal function difficult after a period of injury.

A simple method of producing brain edema involves placing a freezing

Table 9–2. Experimental Methods to Produce Brain Edema

Method	Type of Edema	Reference
Freezing probe to cortex	Vasogenic	Klatzo et al., 1958
Vascular occlusion	Cytotoxic and vasogenic	Levine, 1960
Fluid infusion into CSF	Interstitial	Rosenberg et al., 1983
Intravenous hypotonic solutions	Cytotoxic	Van Harreveld et al., 1966
Triethyltin	Cytotoxic	Katzman et al., 1963
Free radical injection	Vasogenic	Chan et al., 1984

probe on the surface of the skull or on the exposed brain (Klatzo et al., 1965). Cortex is damaged, and vasogenic edema results. Another method involves injection of systemic toxins that injure brain cells. Triethyltin is a toxin that has been used to produce cytotoxic edema (Katzman et al., 1963). Infusion of hypotonic solutions causes cellular swelling, producing an experimental model of cytotoxic edema (Van Harreveld et al., 1966; Wasterlain and Posner, 1968; Wasterlain and Torack, 1968). Direct injection of toxic materials into brain has been used to produce edema. Infusion directly into brain tissue of arachidonic acid and free radical generating systems results in brain edema with disruption of the blood–brain barrier (Chan et al., 1983).

Traumatic edema can be produced in the cortex or the spinal cord by percussion of the tissue. Standardized methods for percussion of the cortex or cord have been developed (McIntosh et al., 1987). The skull or vertebrae are removed, and a standardized weight is dropped onto the dura to cause a reproducible injury.

9.3.2 Vasogenic Edema

An injury to the brain experimentally produced by freezing the cortex damages the blood–brain barrier. Serum proteins, electrolytes, and water enter brain tissue (Klatzo et al., 1965). Fluid leaving the capillary enlarges the extracellular space primarily in the white matter. This results in an increase in water content in white matter, where a high sodium and low potassium content is found (Pappius and Gulati, 1963). The composition of the edema is similar to that of an ultrafiltrate of blood, suggesting that the excess fluid is derived directly from blood. Gray matter is affected by the trauma of freezing at the site of injury, whereas white matter undergoes changes at distant sites.

Transport of substances in the extracellular fluid occurs by diffusion and bulk flow (convection). Diffusion is a random process that depends on the molecular weight and temperature, and bulk flow occurs along osmotic and hydrostatic gradients (Rosenberg et al., 1980). The excess fluid in the edematous brain is transported along white matter fiber tracts and perivascular spaces. There is less movement within the extracellular matrix of the gray matter, which contains a densely interwoven synaptic network (Rosenberg et al., 1983). An important pathway for solute movement appears to be within the perivascular space (Rennels et al., 1985). Bulk flow is an important mechanism for removal from brain of substances of different molecular weights under normal conditions, since diffusion is too slow a process, particularly for larger molecules (Cserr et al., 1981).

Edema fluid moves through brain tissue by bulk flow along pressure gradients (Rosenberg et al., 1978). The highest pressures are found near the injury, and they fall off with distance from the injured area. Radiolabeled sucrose injected intravenously after a cold injury to cat cortex penetrates initially into the white matter near the injured cortex, and with time the extracellular sucrose molecule is seen to spread by bulk flow through the white matter toward the ventricle to drain into the CSF (Reulen et al., 1978). Increased hydrostatic pressure enhances the spread of interstitial fluid. Hypertension enhances the spread of fluid away from the site of injury (Klatzo et al., 1965), and raised CSF pressure enhances the flow into brain (Rosenberg et al., 1982, 1983).

Electron microscopy of vasogenic brain edema has demonstrated an enlarged extracellular space in the white matter, whereas in gray matter, extracellular space is preserved (Long et al., 1966). In vasogenic edema, the primary damage occurs at the blood vessels. Brain tumors and abscesses injure the blood vessels and result in vasogenic edema. Tumors damage the vessel by either outgrowing their blood supply, producing a necrotic center, or secreting substances that increase blood vessel permeability.

Spread of edema fluid in the white matter raises ICP and interferes with CBF. When the ICP exceeds that of the blood, cerebral perfusion pressure is reduced to a level insufficient to maintain oxygenation. Anoxia occurs with tissue damage. Lack of cerebral perfusion leads to brain cell death.

9.3.3 Cytotoxic Edema

Cytotoxic edema occurs from direct damage to brain cells. Hypoxia–ischemia, hypotonic solutions, and toxins result in cytotoxic edema. Hypoxia–ischemia causes cellular swelling when there is failure of the sodium-potassium-ATPase pump from energy loss. As cells increase in size, there is a shift of water from extracellular to intracellular compartments that can occur without a net gain in water.

Hypoxia, produced by substitution of nitrogen for oxygen in inhaled gases, without ischemia does not necessarily produce edema. Cerebral activity measured by EEG is lost after about 30 seconds of anoxia. Although anaerobic conditions lead to the production of lactate, fatty acids, and acidosis, the water and electrolyte content of whole tissue is unaffected at an early stage, indicating that the dysfunction is related to the shifts in cell volume. Cats with prolonged hypoxia followed by survival for several days showed no change in water, sodium, or potassium content in spite of persistent EEG abnormalities (Norris and Pappius, 1970). The effects of hypoxia alone are compounded by systemic acidosis, hypercapnia, and ischemia. Hypoxia produces an increase in CBF, which allows greater oxygen delivery to the tissues.

Edema resulting from carotid occlusion with superimposed hypoxia is characterized by an initial injury to cells, with a secondary disruption of the blood–brain barrier (Levine, 1960; Plum et al., 1963). In prolonged hypoxia–ischemia when cellular metabolism is disrupted, there is mitochondrial swelling, and neurons become vacuolated, pinocytotic vesicles appear in endothelial cells, and extracellular space decreases. However, edema as measured by the increase in water content is a later occurrence associated with tissue necrosis and with the loss of capillary function. Damage to the blood–brain barrier occurs with excessive accumulation of fluid in tissue. This type of cellular edema has small changes in sodium and potassium content. Following 5–10 minutes of carotid occlusion with hypoxia followed by recirculation, the neurons were damaged and the vessels at this early stage appeared to be intact (Levy et al., 1975).

The gerbil is unique in that it has an incomplete circle of Willis. Unilateral carotid occlusion results in a stroke in a significant number of animals. In a study of the effect of 5 minutes of bilateral carotid occlusion in gerbils followed by recirculation for up to 7 days, a biphasic response of the blood–brain barrier was noted (Suzuki et al., 1983a,b). Shortly after recirculation, an increased vascular permeability to HRP was noted in the hippocampus and parts of the basal ganglia. Evans blue, which binds to albumin, did not show exudation at the early stage. Twelve to 24 hours later, there was a second opening of the blood–brain barrier to both tracers. Regional blood flow showed a reactive hyperemia shortly after recirculation, followed by a marked hypoperfusion lasting for 2 days before returning to normal. Late ischemic changes in the hippocampal neurons were noted and correlated with loss of electrical activity.

Although CBF increases transiently shortly after an episode of hypoxia with or without ischemia, the delayed effect is a reduction in blood flow. If the insult is severe, there may be loss of blood flow or the so-called no-reflow phenomenon (Ames et al., 1968). Studies of the relationship between the CBF and metabolism have shown that there is a blood flow threshold below which severe injury and a loss of high-energy phosphates occur. Blood flow below that threshold leads to the development of brain edema (Crockard et al., 1980). In the gerbil with carotid occlusion and reperfusion, the threshold for blood flow below which brain edema occurred was 20 ml/100 g/minute.

Cytotoxic and vasogenic edema are useful terms that primarily describe accumulation of fluid within cells or in the extracellular space. However, they fail to convey the dynamic nature of the changes that are occurring to both cells and blood vessels. At different stages in the progression of both types of edema, elements of one or the other often are present. In the early stages of vasogenic edema, damage to the blood vessel allows serum proteins and electrolytes to enter the interstitial space. The proteins and electrolytes increase the extracellular fluid osmotic pressure, and water follows. Sodium is an important factor in the control of extracellular volume. In the white matter, the extracellular space enlarges. Bulk flow attempts to remove the fluid from the extracellular space, but the increase in extracellular volume raises ICP. At this stage, the edema fluid may compress the blood vessels and lead to compromise of the cerebral circulation.

Cytotoxic edema caused by intracerebral hemorrhage is seen well on CT scan where the blood has high density. Areas of cerebral infarcts often are absent on CT scan for up to 1 week, whereas the MRI scan shows the injured area early in the course. Cerebral hemorrhages were mistakenly diagnosed as infarcts before the use of CT scans. Particularly difficult to diagnose were small hemorrhages with few symptoms. As expected, the greater the size of the hemorrhage, the worse the prognosis (Tuhrim et al., 1988). Small hemorrhages displace less brain tissue and do not result in brain edema. Most likely, the secondary edema and resulting brain ischemia are the cause of the high mortality from hemorrhages. Surgical removal of hemorrhages has been attempted, with limited success, and it is generally not recommended (McKissock et al., 1961).

9.3.4 Interstitial Edema

Interstitial edema refers to the periventricular edema that occurs in hydrocephalus (Fishman, 1975). When the normal mechanism of absorption through the base of the brain and over the convexities is blocked, the excess fluid dilates the ventricles and forces fluid into the periventricular white matter. Transependymal absorption causes enlargement of the extracellular space and, if present for sufficient time, leads to permanent damage to the white matter (Milhorat et al., 1970). The blood–brain barrier remains intact, and the neurons are not affected. Injection of HRP into the ventricle at elevated pressure causes its movement along perivascular spaces and fiber tracts in the white matter (Figure 9–3). Along with the movement into white matter there is an impairment in cerebral blood flow to the periventricular regions (Rosenberg et al., 1983).

The role of the interstitial fluid in the development of pathological lesions is poorly understood. Several possible mechanisms exist for tissue to be damaged, but experimental verification is lacking at this time. One potential mechanism is congestion of the perivascular spaces, with prevention of the removal of toxic metabolites and neurotransmitters, such as glutamate and the phospholipases. The edema fluid could prevent movement of fluid along this route. More likely, however, is that the movement of interstitial fluid from the cerebral ventricles to brain prevents the normal drainage of interstitial fluid into the CSF. By interfering with the lymph-like role of interstitial fluid, the abnormal flow patterns result in tissue damage.

9.4 HYDROCEPHALUS

Hydrocephalus is a common cause of interstitial edema. Patients with hydrocephalus have reduced CBF to the periventricular areas (Greitz et al., 1969). The blood flow can return to normal after treatment by draining the excess fluid from the ventricle through a tube placed in the ventricle to drain into the heart or abdominal cavity. The MRI in hydrocephalus shows periventricular fluid with a halo around the ventricle, but prediction of benefit from treatment by MRI is difficult (Figure 9–4). Both CT and MRI are excellent modalities to determine ventricular enlargement. The MRI, however, is better in distinguishing transependymal fluid movement than is CT scan.

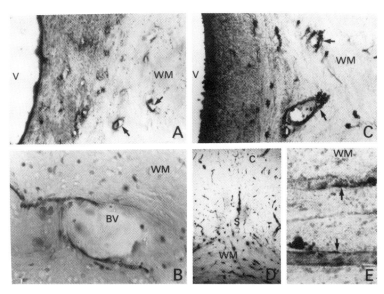

Figure 9–3. Photomicrographs from animals after ventriculocisternal perfusions with horseradish peroxidase (HRP) at various pressures for 4 hours. A. Sample after control perfusion at −5 cm H₂O pressure. A section of the ventricle (V) is shown with adjacent white matter (WM). The ependyma is densely stained with HRP reaction product, with some penetration into the white matter. Several blood vessels are seen surrounded by HRP (arrows). ×7. B. High-power view of a blood vessel (BV) in the white matter several millimeters from the surface in a control animal. Staining by HRP is absent. ×28. C. Sample after high-pressure perfusion with HRP, showing an area similar to that illustrated in A. There is increased penetration of the HRP reaction product into the white matter, particularly around blood vessels (arrows). ×7. D. Low-power view of deep white matter in the sulcus of the cortex (C) in a high-pressure perfusion sample. The white matter including that penetrating into the cortical sulcus (S) shows dense accumulation of HRP reaction product. Again, blood vessels are well visualized. ×1.75. E. An area of deep white matter corresponding to B, with several blood vessles (arrows) in a high-pressure perfusion sample. Diffuse staining of the white matter is seen. ×28. (From Rosenberg et al., 1983)

Hydrocephalus is divided into communicating and noncommunicating forms. Communicating implies an open connection between the fourth ventricle and the subarachnoid space, and noncommunicating is used to describe a blockage before the ventricular outflow pathways. The site of outflow obstruction can be at the arachnoid villi or the base of the brain in the communicating forms. Substances injected into the lumbar CSF can pass into the ventricles in communicating hydrocephalus, whereas intraventricular injection is required for substances to enter the ventricles in the noncommunicating forms.

There are multiple causes of hydrocephalus. Subarachnoid hemorrhage and meningitis are frequent causes, and masses and congenital anomalies are less common. Blood in the subarachnoid space clogs the arachnoid villi, producing a transient ventricular enlargement. A small percentage of patients

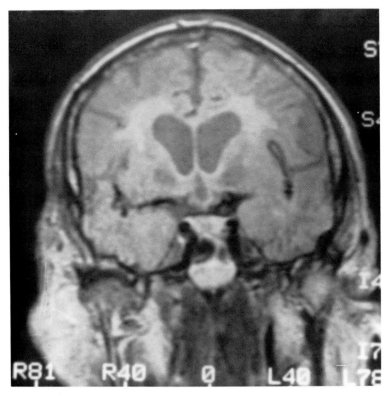

Figure 9–4. MRI scan from patient with normal pressure hydrocephalus. Inter-mediate-weighted image shows fluid (white) around the ventricles (dark) and in the frontal white matter.

go on to develop hydrocephalus. Fungal meningitis can produce chronic hy-drocephalus.

Hydrocephalus of the noncommunicating type tends to evolve more rap-idly, often with life-threatening symptoms. Communicating hydrocephalus develops more slowly. A classification based on clinical course is given in Table 9–3. Since all forms of hydrocephalus are by definition obstructive, the course depends mainly on the development of alternative absorptive mechanisms. The age of the patient and the rapidity of the ventricular en-largement are factors that determine the clinical course.

Isotope cisternography shows reflux of isotope into the ventricles in nor-mal pressure hydrocephalus with ventricular persistence for over 24 hours. Cisternography is done by injection of a technetium-labeled substance into the lumbar sac. Normally, all of the gamma-emitter passes over the con-vexity by 24 hours (Figure 9–5). In ventricles enlarged because of atrophy, the tracer enters the ventricles, but it is removed by 48 hours (DiChiro et al., 1964). When there is transependymal flow, the tracer enters the ventricle and remains there for over 48 hours (Benson et al., 1970). An example of persistent ventricular filling is shown in Figure 9–6.

Table 9–3. Clinical Classification of Hydrocephalic Syndromes

Acute or Subacute	Chronic
Intraventricular mass	Posthemorrhagic
Colloid cyst	Subarachnoid hemorrhage
Tumor	Trauma/surgery
Posterior fossa mass	Postinfectious
Tumor	Bacterial
Hematoma/infarct	Fungal
Aqueductal stenosis	Viral
Ventriculitis	Arnold-Chiari malformation
Bacterial	Excessive CSF protein
Viral	Tumor
Developmental abnormalities	Guillain-Barré syndrome
Aqueductal stenosis	Overproduction of CSF
Dandy-Walker syndrome	Agenesis of the arachnoid villi
	Idiopathic (normal-pressure)

Infusion of fluid into the subarachnoid space has been done experimentally in people, increasing ICP without cerebral symptoms (Foldes et al., 1948). A normal person can tolerate the infusion of moderate amounts of artificial CSF or normal saline, with the CSF pressure reaching a new plateau (Katzman et al., 1970). In patients with disorders of CSF absorption, the resistance to outflow can be tested clinically with an infusion test (Hussey and Katzman, 1970). This test has been used to determine the resistance to CSF outflow in patients with suspected normal-pressure hydrocephalus (NPH). The test has been modified by several investigators and is used in

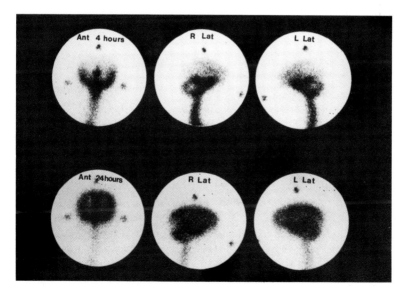

Figure 9–5. Normal cisternogram. The radiolabeled tracer was injected into the lumbar sac and is seen at 4 and 24 hours in the cisterna and over the convexity, respectively. None of the tracer appears in the ventricles. (Courtesy of Dr. F. A. Mettler, Jr.)

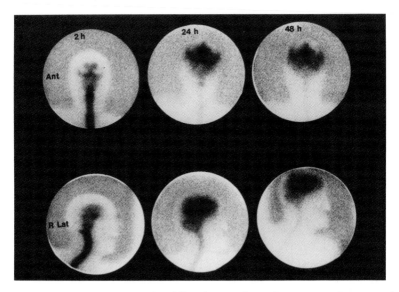

Figure 9–6. Persistent ventricular filling is seen in a cisternogram from a patient with normal pressure hydrocephalus. The tracer injected into the lumbar sac enters the ventricles and persists for over 48 hours. (Courtesy of Dr. F. A. Mettler, Jr.)

some centers as a diagnostic tool. The clinical usefulness is limited because negative tests can occur in individuals with NPH in whom alternate drainage pathways for the removal of CSF have developed.

A clinical syndrome of gait disturbance, urinary incontinence, and dementia in elderly patients has been associated with occult hydrocephalus (Adams et al., 1965). The symptoms begin insidiously in most patients without a clear etiology. Some patients with the syndrome of NPH have a history of meningitis or subarachnoid hemorrhage. When the symptoms are gait disturbance and incontinence, the response to surgical placement of a shunt is improved. The search for a diagnostic test in NPH has not been successful, and assessment of the clinical situation is needed. In general, those individuals with long-standing symptoms, prominent dementia, and mild gait problems respond least well to surgical treatment. However, there is no medical treatment for this progressive illness, and shunt placement is used as a last resort.

Thirty to fifty percent of patients with NPH have an associated illness as the cause, and in the remainder, the NPH is termed idiopathic because a cause is lacking. In spite of numerous studies of the CSF dynamics in NPH, the relationship among ventricular enlargement, pressure–volume index, and response to shunting is highly variable (Tans and Poortvliet, 1988). A global defect in cerebral glucose metabolism has been found in 3 patients with NPH by PET scanning (Jagust et al., 1985). Until an accurate diagnostic test is available, selection of patients with occult hydrocephalus for shunting will remain empirical.

There is an increasing awareness of the connection between hypertensive vascular disease of the white matter, or so-called Binswanger's disease, and NPH (Figure 9–7). A relationship between hypertensive lacunar state and NPH has been reported (Earnest et al., 1974; Koto et al., 1977). MRI has revealed a high incidence of increased proton signals in the white matter in people with hypertension. Some of these individuals have cerebral symptoms, whereas others do not.

Considerable controversy has developed over the significance of increased proton signals from the white matter that are seen commonly on MRI in patients with multiple strokes, Alzheimer's disease, hydrocephalus, collagen vascular diseases, viral infection, and trauma. The appearance of these lesions is similar to those seen in patients with demyelination due to multiple sclerosis. The problem is that they are found in some otherwise normal elderly people, particularly those with hypertension (Steingart et al., 1987a,b; Hunt et al., 1989). Pathological studies in normal individuals with white matter lesions have shown a high incidence of blood vessel fibrosis from hypertension, with an increased interstitial space (Awad et al., 1986). In patients with diffuse demyelination due to Binswanger's disease, the same vascular changes are observed pathologically, but they are less extensive (Olzewski, 1965; Rosenberg et al., 1979). The etiology of vascular forms of demyelination is thought to be ischemia (Inzitari et al., 1987), but the underlying cause of the white matter changes remains to be determined.

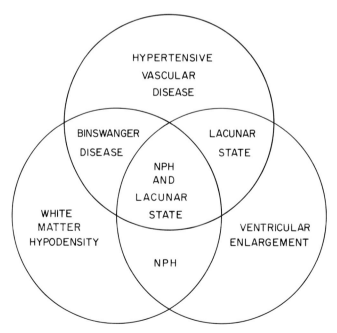

Figure 9–7. Venn diagram illustrating overlapping of patients with hypertensive vascular disease, white matter hypodensity on CT, and enlarged ventricles.

9.5 IRREVERSIBLE METABOLIC EVENTS WITH EDEMA

Prolonged ischemia with recirculation produces a series of metabolic changes (Siesjo and Wieloch, 1985). PCr levels rapidly fall to zero in an attempt to form ATP from excess ADP. Lactate rises to reach a plateau, ATP levels decrease to zero, and free fatty acids are formed. After restoration of circulation, PCr rises and overshoots, energy charge follows closely, and lactate and free fatty acids gradually return to normal.

^{31}P-NMR and ^{1}H-NMR has been used to measure in vivo pH and brain lactate in injured tissue. Although lactate may correlate with pH in some circumstances, there is at times a dissociation between lactate levels and cellular pH (Paschen et al., 1987). This suggests other causes for the acidosis, such as ATP hydrolysis. Removal of excess acid depends on bicarbonate and on sodium. Sodium is cotransported with protons. In hyponatremic animals with acidosis due to hypercapnia, there is a greater reduction in pH than in normonatremic animals (Adler, 1989). This may be because of the inability to remove H^+ in the absence of Na^+ (Figure 9–8). In brain trauma, the severity of the brain injury has been shown by ^{31}P-NMR and ^{1}H-NMR to correlate with the fall in pH and with lactate build-up in the injured area (McIntosh et al., 1987).

9.6 BRAIN LIPIDS IN EDEMA

There is increasing evidence that irreversible damage to the cell results when the membrane is attacked during lipid peroxidation. Membrane phospholipids contain polyunsaturated fatty acids (PUFAs) attached to glyerol at the C2 position. Linoleic acid ($C_{18:2}$) and linolenic acid ($C_{18:4}$) are essential in the diet but can be elongated in the body to arachidonic acid ($C_{20:4}$) and docosahexenoic acid ($C_{22:6}$), respectively. These two PUFAs increase in both ischemia and severe hypoxia (Barzan, 1970; Gardiner et al., 1981; Yoshida et al., 1982). Release of fatty acids occurs by activation of the phospholipases. With the loss of energy substrate, the ability to resynthesize phospholipids is impaired. The fatty acids released have both a direct toxic action on brain cells and an indirect action through the formation of prostaglandins, leukotrienes, and free radicals.

Arachidonic acid alters the packing of lipid molecules, increases membrane fluidity, stimulates chloride transport in corneal epithelium, and enhances activity of adenylate cyclase and guanylate cyclase (Usher et al., 1978; Schaeffer and Zadunaisky, 1979; Wallach and Pastan, 1976). Arachidonic acid and free-radical generating solutions induced edema when applied to cortical slices or injected directly into brain (Chan et al., 1983, 1984, 1985).

Although arachidonic acid and other free fatty acids are toxic in themselves, the products of their degeneration further enhance their toxicity. Formation of reactive oxygen metabolites that rapidly oxidize biological mol-

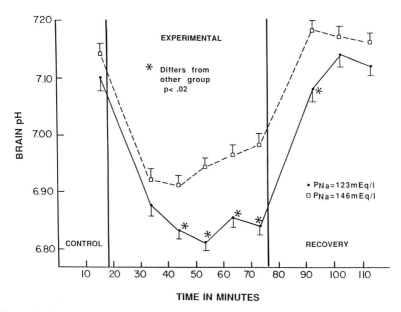

Figure 9–8. Rats exposed to 20 percent CO_2, 30 percent O_2, and 50 percent N_2O during experimental period. ^{31}P-NMR with surface coils was used to record in vivo spectra for calculation of brain pH. Hyponatremic animals had a lower pH than had normonatremic animals. During the control and recovery periods, animals received 30 percent O_2 and 70 percent N_2O. (From Adler, 1989)

ecules appears to be an important process in irreversible cell damage. These highly reactive substances are called "free radicals," since they contain unpaired electrons. Normally, the 4-electron reduction of O_2 to form H_2O proceeds by a well-controlled mechanism in the mitochondrial electron transport system that requires cytochrome oxidase. The production of reduced oxygen species is written as

$$O_2 + e^- \rightarrow O_2^- \cdot \text{ (superoxide)} \tag{9–1}$$

$$O_2 + 2e^- + 2H^+ \rightarrow H_2O_2 \text{ (hydrogen peroxide)} \tag{9–2}$$

$$O_2^- \cdot + H_2O_2 + H^+ \rightarrow O_2 + H_2O + OH \cdot \text{ (hydroxyl radical)} \tag{9–3}$$

$$O_2 + 4e^- + 4H^+ \rightarrow 2H_2O \text{ (water)} \tag{9–4}$$

The superoxide ($O_2^- \cdot$), hydrogen peroxide (H_2O_2), and hydroxyl radical ($OH \cdot$) are toxic species.

Iron is important as a catalyst for hydroxyl radical formation, by the Haber-Weiss reactions.

$$O_2^- \cdot + Fe^{3+} \rightarrow O_2 + Fe^{2+} \tag{9–5}$$

$$H_2O_2 + Fe^{2+} \rightarrow HO^{\cdot} + OH^- + Fe^{3+} \qquad (9-6)$$

$$Sum: O_2^{-\cdot} + H_2O_2 \rightarrow HO^{\cdot} + OH^- + O_2 \qquad (9-7)$$

The reduction of ferric to ferrous iron by $O_2^{-\cdot}$ begins the process, which requires hydrogen peroxide formation from the superoxide radical. The $HO^{\cdot}$ is the most reactive oxygen species found in biological systems.

Lipid peroxidation occurs when $HO^{\cdot}$ removes methylene hydrogen atoms from PUFAs. The reaction of $HO^{\cdot}$ with polyunsaturated fatty acids is

$$LH + HO^{\cdot} \rightarrow H_2O + L^{\cdot} \qquad (9-8)$$

$$L^{\cdot} + O_2 \rightarrow LOO^{\cdot} \qquad (9-9)$$

$$LOO^{\cdot} + LH \rightarrow LOOH + L^{\cdot} \qquad (9-10)$$

$$L^{\cdot} + L^{\cdot} \rightarrow L-L \qquad (9-11)$$

where LH, $L^{\cdot}$, $LOO^{\cdot}$, and LOOH represent polyunsaturated lipid, lipid aklyl radical, lipid perhydroxyl radical, and lipid hydroperoxide, respectively (Grisham and McCord, 1986). The cytotoxicity of free radicals is thought to be due to the peroxidation of membrane-associated polyunsaturated fatty acids by $HO^{\cdot}$ with lysis of the cell (Stocks and Dormandy, 1971). Neutrophils form free radical species that activate latent collagenases that may be important in neutrophil-mediated cytotoxicity (Weiss et al., 1985).

There are endogenous antioxidant enzymes and free radical scavengers that protect cells from the action of reactive O_2 metabolites. Superoxide dismutase catalyzes the production of H_2O_2 from $O_2^{-\cdot}$, and catalase promotes the formation of O_2 and H_2O from H_2O_2. These enzymes prevent the formation of highly reactive $HO^{\cdot}$ and hypochlorous acid (HOCl). The second level of defense is the scavengers, such as alpha-tocopherol (vitamin E) and mannitol (Grisham and McCord, 1986). The enzyme superoxide dismutase is found normally inside the cell membrane. Superoxide dismutase can be incorporated into liposomes and introduced into cells to protect them against oxidation (Turrens et al., 1984).

There are free radical-generating systems based on the oxidation of hypoxanthine by xanthine oxidase. Infusion of a free radical-generating system into brain resulted in edema formation (Chan et al., 1984). When these investigators infused liposome-encapsulated superoxide dismutase into animals with cold-injured cortex, they found a reduction in the edema formation (Chan et al., 1987).

There are two potential sources of free radicals in brain, namely, the xanthines and the arachidonic acid catabolic cascade, that are important in cell damage. Membranes in brain cells contain PUFAs that are released by lipases. Arachidonic acid released from membranes is metabolized by cyclooxygenase and lipoxygenase to form reactive oxygen species. For free radicals to be formed, some oxygen is necessary. This is probably the reason that, in ischemia, the tissue damage occurs mainly during reperfusion when oxygen is again available. Xanthines produce free radicals during nucleotide metabolism. When ATP is converted to ADP, the nucleotides, adenosine, inosine, and hypoxanthine, are formed. Xanthine dehydrogenase is converted to xanthine oxidase by Ca^{2+}-dependent proteases that occur when Ca^{2+} enters cells. Finally, the xanthine oxidase converts hypoxanthine into a free radical in the presence of oxygen (Siesjo and Wieloch, 1985). Whether xanthine metabolism or the arachidonic cascade is the primary mechanism of tissue peroxidation during brain injury remains to be established.

9.7 TREATMENT OF BRAIN EDEMA

Osmotherapy is the most effective treatment for vasogenic and cytotoxic brain edema (Table 9–1). Initially, hyperosmolar solutions of urea were used, but since urea enters cells, the osmotic effect was lost with time, and there often was a rebound increase in pressure (Bering, 1960). The nonmetabolized sugar, mannitol, which is normally prevented from entering brain by the blood–brain barrier, is the current agent of choice (Wise and Chater, 1962). When mannitol was first introduced into clinical practice, the recommended dosage ranged from 2 to 3 g/kg, which was thought to be necessary to remove water from brain tissue. However, at that dose, the agent could be given only one or two times in a 12–24 hour period because of the electrolyte disturbances associated with the resulting diuresis. Currently, much lower amounts of mannitol in the range of 0.25 to 1 g/kg are recommended, and these doses lower ICP without affecting electrolytes (Marshall et al., 1978). With the lower amounts, it has been possible to control raised ICP over several days.

Tissue dehydration occurs when serum osmolality increases over 30 mOsm/ kg (Stern and Coxon, 1964). Water is removed from normal tissue, since the disrupted blood–brain barrier prevents the development of an osmotic gradient. Mannitol reduces CSF formation (Sahar and Tsipsteln, 1978), which contributes to its ability to lower ICP. The rebound increase in CSF pressure occasionally seen with urea is very rare with mannitol. Mannitol is unique among the group of hyperosmolar agents that have been tried clinically, including urea and glycerol, in that it does not increase the osmolality of the CSF. Therefore, there is an osmotic gradient between the brain and the CSF that favors movement of CSF into brain (Rosenberg et al., 1980; Cserr et al., 1987; Pullen et al., 1987). This bulk flow into brain is thought to compensate for fluid lost to the hyperosmolar blood in order to preserve brain volume.

Steroids are used to treat brain edema. They are most effective in edema associated with brain tumors. The usefulness of steroids, even in large doses, in the treatment of edema due to ischemia or head injury is controversial.

In some circumstances, such as edema secondary to cerebral malaria, they may be harmful (Warrell et al., 1982). A large retrospective study of the use of steroids in acute ischemic strokes showed no benefit (De Reuck et al., 1988). The mechanism of action of steroids is not known. They influence water balance in a complex manner. For example, they have been shown to be helpful in lowering ICP in pseudotumor cerebri. However, when their use is stopped, they can cause a temporary increase in pressure. Dexamethasone, the most commonly used agent, affects the immune response and inhibits brain enzymes, such as plasminogen activator (Levin and Los-Kutoff, 1982; Roblin and Young, 1980). A high correlation exists between levels of plasminogen activator activity in brain tumors and perineoplastic edema on CT (Quindlen and Bucher, 1987). Another potentially important action of glucocorticoids is to induce the synthesis of proteins that inhibit phospholipase A_2 (Blackwell et al., 1980).

Other agents have been used experimentally in edema treatment. High doses of barbiturates reduce cellular metabolism and, in some experimental studies, were effective in treatment of edema. However, clinical tests have been unable to show a beneficial effect of barbiturate-induced coma in head trauma or cardiac arrest (Brain Resuscitation Study Group, 1986). Agents that block free radical formation or are free radical scavengers have been used experimentally, but their usefulness in patients has not been proven.

9.8 RECOVERY OF FUNCTION AFTER BRAIN INJURY

The goal of treatment in brain edema is to reduce the brain swelling to prevent the secondary damage resulting from loss of blood flow and hypoxia. The maximum swelling in acute injuries occurs at 24–48 hours. Deterioration in clinical status within this time frame generally indicates the presence of edema. The brain swelling leads to shifts of brain tissue that compress the tissue on to various bony or hard collagenous structures. The shift of brain tissue is referred to as "herniation." For example, lesions in the temporal lobe compress the structures in the midbrain against the tentorium. Shifts of the frontal lobes across the midline and of the cerebellum through the foramen also can occur.

Edema caused by brain tumors is less consistent. Some tumors, such as the oligodendrogliomas, whose cellular composition is similar to that of brain, cause little edema and produce symptoms as a result of their size and location. However, metastatic tumors cause extensive brain edema, which usually responds well to steroid treatment.

After the acute phase of the cerebral insult has passed, a gradual recovery of function can occur. In head-injured patients, the recovery depends on multiple factors, including extent of the initial injury, age of the patient, and other injuries. Younger patients recover better than older ones for reasons that are unclear but must be studied. Secondary factors, such as hypotension, fat emboli from long bone fractures, and abdominal injuries with circulating pancreatic enzymes, affect the eventual recovery. Although full recovery from severe head injury may not occur, some patients have regained function even after a prolonged vegetative state. The severity of the injuries has limited the amount of information available about brain metabolism in these patients.

Recovery from stroke has been studied intensely. The TIAs improve by definition by 24 hours, and most patients regain function within 10 minutes. Longer periods of ischemia result in permanent injury to tissue. When the neurological deficit lasts over 24 hours, it is generally considered to be a cerebral infarction. The rate of recovery depends on several factors: the extent of the ischemic insult, the age of the patient, and the presence of other illnesses, including diabetes mellitus and hypertension. Because of the large numbers of people with head injury or stroke, there is great interest in the mechanisms of recovery.

9.9 OVERVIEW AND POTENTIAL TREATMENTS

Activation of edema-forming processes occurs after many different types of brain damage. Although these multiple factors have been discussed separately, in reality they are occurring simultaneously and interacting to worsen the resulting edema. Figure 9–9 shows the cascade of interlocking events along with potential therapeutic interventions. Some of the events shown in Figure 9–9 occur earlier than others, suggesting that the therapeutic window for each drug will be different. Calcium channel blockers are useful only in the early phases of the acute injury and ideally would be given before the injury, which is not feasible. Inhibitors of free fatty acid breakdown would probably be best given in the later stages of the injury when the various reaction products are being formed, whereas other agents, such as amphetamines, are effective in enhancing recovery when given days after the injury.

Long-term recovery studies are difficult to perform in either animals or patients. Grading scales have been developed to assess recovery of function in animals; the acute injuries are subject to variability. A single end-point of death fails to detect small but still significant improvement after a given treatment. Human studies are complicated by the need to obtain similar groups of patients in the face of highly variable clinical conditions. Stroke studies have evaluated time to recover function and death, but finding patients with comparable lesions can be very difficult. The various exclusion criteria for drug studies are generally stringent, leading to a further reduction in numbers of patients available for study in a single center. Multicenter collaborative studies have been used to overcome some of the difficulties.

A number of agents have been shown to reduce brain damage after various insults (Table 9–4). Opioid antagonists have been shown to improve recovery after spinal cord injury (Faden et al., 1981) and after stroke (Hosobuchi et al., 1982). Studies with naloxone in cerebral ischemia have produced

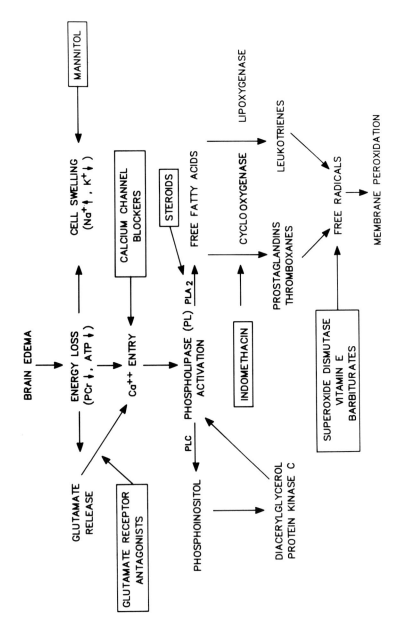

Figure 9–9. Schematic diagram of the multiple interacting events in the evolution of brain edema. The boxes indicate potential sites of therapeutic intervention. PCr, phosphocreatinine; PLC, phospholipase C; PLA$_2$, phospholipase A$_2$.

Table 9–4. Experimental Agents to Reduce Brain Damage

Agent	Mechanism of Action
Naloxone	Opioid receptor antagonist
Ganglioside GM_1	Na^+,K^+-ATPase preserved
Amphetamines	Effect on biogenic amines
Platelet activating factor inhibitor	Decrease Ca^{2+} influx
Thyrotropin-releasing hormone (TRH)	Opioid antagonist

conflicting results, possibly because of the complex actions of naloxone on CBF and the need to use high doses of the drug, which may affect nonopioid-mediated functions. Gangliosides have been shown in experimental ischemia to reduce the extent of tissue injury (Karpiak et al., 1987). Gangliosides are thought to act by protecting membranes from loss of Na^+, K^+-ATPase; it was necessary to give these agents shortly after the injury. In animals with open head injury, gangliosides were found to reduce edema (Karpiak and Mahadik, 1984). Stabilization of membranes has been proposed to reduce lipid hydrolysis, lipase activation, and arachidonic acid release.

Enhancement of recovery in injured rats and cats was produced by the administration of amphetamines (Feeney et al., 1982). Rats given a single dose of amphetamine 1 day after an injury to the motor cortex recovered faster than did untreated, injured rats. The animals had to be handled; therefore, an experience factor also was involved. The hypothesis that amphetamine along with physical therapy would improve function was tested in a small group of stroke patients, and amphetamine was found to be beneficial (Crisostomo et al., 1987).

A naturally occurring alkyl-ether phospholipid, platelet-activating factor (PAF), is a potent activator of platelets and a mediator of the inflammatory process. In neuronal cell lines, PAF was found to increase the uptake of Ca^{2+} from the extracellular environment. The uptake was blocked by a PAF antagonist and by calcium channel blockers (Kornecki and Ehrlich, 1988). A possible mechanism of PAF pathogenesis was shown in neurons, where the increased levels of Ca^{2+} could lead to activation of phospholipase A_2 and release of free PUFAs (Panetta et al., 1987). PAF antagonists occur in nature in extracts of the *Ginkgo biloba* tree. Several ginkolides have been tested for a protective effect against ischemia in the gerbil vessel-occlusion model, and the ginkolide, BN 52021, had the greatest protective effect. Other PAF antagonists, kadsurenone and brotizolam, also are effective in ischemia (Spinnewyn et al., 1987).

Thyrotropin-releasing hormone (TRH) has been found to reduce the extent of spinal cord injury in rabbits (Faden et al., 1981). The TRH acts in a similar fashion to opioid antagonists in that it improves spinal cord blood flow, reduces pathological changes, and improves long-term outcome. These agents show promise in spinal cord-injured patients and are under clinical investigation.

9.10 EPILOGUE

Neurotransmitters and neuropeptides amplify and modulate the signals between brain cells. There exists a large number of such substances, and the list continues to grow. The large number of amplifiers and modulators that are found in mammals may explain the increasing complexity of their nervous systems in spite of similarities between mammals in brain structure. However, the complexity of communication mechanisms of brain cells, which in a sense act as amplifiers of neural signals, also may provide a framework for cellular disruption. The reason for this is that a normal signal when activated to excessive activity could trigger a sequence of events that amplify the response, resulting in damage to the cell. An overabundance of neurotransmitters and modulators in a specific region, as found in the hippocampus, would make those regions more vulnerable to self-destruction once the damage was underway.

The abundance of substances within the cell that have the potential to destroy the cell is a curious feature of evolution. Glutamate, calcium, lysosomal enzymes, and arachidonic acid are all normal components of cells that have the potential to destroy the cell. Most glutamate used normally in energy generation is compartmentalized into biochemically inaccessible compartments separated from the neurotransmitter pool of glutamate. Calcium is sequestered in mitochondria and endoplasmic reticulum. Lysosomal enzymes are contained within vesicles of very low pH. Even normally present ions, such as chloride and potassium, may become toxic. Chloride enters cells after excessive glutamate stimulation to cause cellular swelling; potassium in excessive extracellular amounts depolarizes the cell. Second messengers released by receptor stimulation in normal concentrations lead to cell membrane changes, but with excessive stimulation, they activate pathological processes.

Because of the complexity of these systems, they have had to be analyzed separately. Although this has helped to increase our understanding of the basic mechanisms, it has obscured the interaction and amplification of these reactions. It is difficult to see the evolutionary benefits of these reactions except that they may have begun as scavenger reactions to combat the entry of foreign matter. The organism would sacrifice some of its own cells to help kill the offending invader. This mechanism has been triggered by other than foreign substances. In the case of a cerebral hemorrhage, removal of the debris is accomplished by the scavenger cells. Unfortunately, in the scavenger process, substances are released in the vicinity of normal cells that lead to their overreacting, swelling, and possibly dying.

Damping of the amplifying signals that are destroying normal cells while permitting the scavenger function of cells collecting debris is necessary to provide a framework for recovery. The strategies that have been used vary from surgical removal of the necrotic or hemorrhagic tissue, as in brain trauma or intracerebral hemorrhage, to attempts to block secondary edema formation and to reduce raised pressure with osmotic agents.

The future of therapeutic intervention depends on our ability to have an impact on the multiple systems and to combine therapeutic interventions to combat early and late consequences of brain damage. Important advances have been made in the increasingly large numbers of drugs that interfere with the cascade of cell damage and the increasingly sophisticated in vivo measuring devices that permit us to follow the events over time. The challenge remains, however, to test these agents singly and in combination in closely monitored patients, with the ultimate goal of improving survival while maintaining quality of life.

REFERENCES

Adams, R. D., Fischer, C. M., Hakin, S., Ojemann, R. G., Sweet, W. H.: Symptomatic occult hydrocephalus with "normal" cerebrospinal fluid pressure. N. Engl. J. Med. 273:117–126, 1965.

Adler, S., Simplaceanu, V.: Effect of acute hyponatremia on rat brain pH and rat brain buffering. Am. J. Physiol. 256:F113–F119, 1989.

Ames, A., Wright, R. L., Kowada, M., Thurston, J. M., Majno, G.: Cerebral ischemia. II. The no-reflow phenomenon. Am. J. Pathol. 52:437–453, 1968.

Awad, I. A., Johnson, P. C., Spetzler, R. F., Hodak, J. A.: Incidental subcortical lesions identified on magnetic resonance imaging in the elderly. II. Post-mortem pathological correlations. Stroke 17:1090–1097, 1986.

Bazán, N. G., Jr.: Effects of ischemia and electroconvulsive shock on free fatty acid pool in the brain. Biochim. Biophys. Acta. 218:1–10, 1970.

Benson, D. F., LeMay, M., Patten, D. H., Rubens, A. B.: Diagnosis of normal-pressure hydrocephalus. N. Engl. J. Med. 283:609–615, 1970.

Bering, E. A., Jr., Avman, N.: The use of hypertonic urea solutions in hypothermia. J. Neurosurg. 17:1073–1082, 1960.

Blackwell, G. J., Carnuccio, R., Di Rosa, M., Flower, R. J., Parente, L., Persico, P.: Macrocortin: A polypeptide causing the anti-phospholipase effect of glucocorticoids. Nature 287:147–149, 1980.

Brain Resuscitation Clinical Trial I Study Group: Randomized clinical study of thiopental loading in comatose survivors of cardiac arrest. N. Engl. J. Med. 314:397–403, 1986.

Chan, P. H., Fishman, R. A., Caronna, J., Schmidley, J. W., Prioleau, G., Lee, J.: Induction of brain edema following intracerebral injection of arachidonic acid. Ann. Neurol. 13:625–632, 1983.

Chan, P. H., Fishman, R. A., Longar, S., Chen, S., Yu, A.: Cellular and molecular effects of polyunsaturated fatty acids in brain ischemia and injury. Prog. Brain Res. 63:227–235, 1985.

Chan, P. H., Longar, S., Fishman, R. A.: Protective effects of liposome-entrapped superoxide dismutase on posttraumatic brain edema. Ann. Neurol. 21:540–547, 1987.

Chan, P. H., Schmidley, J. W., Fishman, R. A., Longar, S. M.: Brain injury, edema, and vascular permeability changes induced by oxygen-derived free radicals. Neurology 34:315–320, 1984.

Crisostomo, E. A., Duncan, P. W., Propst, M., Dawson, D. V., Davis, J. N.: Evidence that amphetamine with physical therapy promotes recovery of motor function in stroke patients. Ann. Neurol. 23:94–97, 1988.

Crockard, A., Iannotti, F., Hunstock, A. T., Smith, R. D., Harris, R. J., Symon, L.: Cerebral blood flow and edema following carotid occlusion in the gerbil. Stroke 11:494–498, 1980.

Cserr, H. F., Cooper, D. N., Suri, P. K., Patlak, C. S.: Efflux of radiolabeled polyethylene glycols and albumin from rat brain. Am. J. Physiol. 240:F319–F328, 1981.

Cserr, H. F., DePasquale, M., Patlak, C. S.: Volume regulatory influx of electrolytes from plasma to brain during acute hyperosmolality. Am. J. Physiol. 253:F530–F537, 1987.

Davson, H.: *Physiology of the Cerebrospinal Fluid.* London: Churchill, 1967.

De Reuck, J., Van de Kerckhove, T., Bosma, G., De Meulemeester, K., Van Landegem, W., De Waele, J., Tack, E., De Koninck, J.: Steroid treatment in acute ischaemic stroke. Eur. Neurol. 28:70–72, 1988.

Di Chiro, G., Reames, P. M., Matthews, W. B., Jr.: RISA-ventriculography and RISA-cisternography. Neurology 14:185–191, 1964.

Earnest, M. P., Fahn, S., Karp, J. H., Rowland, L. P.: Normal-pressure hydrocephalus and hypertensive cerebrovascular disease. Arch. Neurol. 31:262–266, 1974.

Faden, A. I., Jacobs, T. P., Holaday, J. W.: Opiate antagonist improves neurologic recovery after spinal injury. Science 211:493–494, 1981.

Feeney, D. M., Gonzales, A., Law, W. A.: Amphetamine, haloperidol, and experience interact to affect rate of recovery after motor cortex injury. Science 217:855–857, 1982.

Fishman, R. A.: Brain edema. N. Engl. J. Med. 293:706–711, 1975.

Foldes, F. F., Arrowood, J. G.: Changes in cerebrospinal fluid pressure under the influence of continuous infusion of normal saline. J. Clin. Invest. 27:346–351, 1948.

Gardiner, M., Nilsson, B., Rehncrona, S., Siesjo, B. K.: Free fatty acids in the rat brain in moderate and severe hypoxia. J. Neurochem. 36:1500–1505, 1981.

Greitz, T. V., Grepe, A. O., Kalmer, M. S., Lopez, J.: Pre- and postoperative evaluation of cerebral blood flow in low-pressure hydrocephalus. J. Neurosurg. 31:644–651, 1969.

Grisham, M. B., McCord, J.: Chemistry and cytotoxicity of reactive oxygen metabolites. In: *Physiology of Oxygen Radicals* (Taylor, A. E., Matalon, A., Ward, P., eds.) Bethesda, Maryland: American Physiological Society, 1980.

Hosobuchi, Y., Baskin D. S., Woo, S. K.: Reversal of induced ischemic neurologic deficit in gerbils by the opiate antagonist naloxone. Science 215:69–71, 1982.

Hunt, A. L., Orrison, W. W., Yeo, R. A., Haaland, K. Y., Rhyne, R. L., Garry, P. J., Rosenberg, G. A.: Clinical significance of MRI white matter lesions in the elderly. Neurology 39:1470–1473. 1989.

Hussey, F., Schanzer, B., Katzman, R.: A simple constant-infusion manometric test for measurement of CSF absorption. II. Clinical studies. Neurology 20:665–680, 1970.

Inzitari, D., Diaz, F., Fox, A., Hachinski, V. C., Steingart, A., Lau, C., Donald, A., Wade, J., Mulic, H., Merskey, H.: Vascular risk factors and leuko-araiosis. Arch. Neurol. 44:42–47, 1987.

Jaqust, W. J., Friedland, R. P., Budinger, T. F.: Positron emission tomography with [18F]fluorodeoxyglucose differentiates normal pressure hydrocephalus from Alzheimer-type dementia. J. Neurol. Neurosurg. Psychiatry 48:1091–1096, 1985.

Karpiak, S. E., Li, Y. S., Mahadik, S. P.: Gangliosides (G_{MI} and AGF2) reduce mortality due to ischemia: Protection of membrane function. Stroke 18:184–187, 1987.

Karpiak, S. E., Mahadik, S. P.: Reduction of cerebral edema with G_{MI} ganglioside. J. Neurosci. Res. 12:485–492, 1984.

Katzman, R., Aleu, F., Wilson, C.: Further observations on triethyl tin edema. Arch. Neurol. 9:178–187, 1963.

Katzman, R., Hussey, F.: A simple constant-infusion manometric test for measurement of CSF absorption. I. Rationale and method. Neurology 20:534–544, 1970.

Klatzo, I.: Presidential Address. Neuropathological aspects of brain edema. J. Neuropathol. Exp. Neurol. 26:1–14, 1967.

Klatzo, I., Piraux, A., Laskowski, E. J.: The relationship between edema, blood–brain barrier and tissue elements in a local brain injury. J. Neuropathol. Exp. Neurol. 17:546–548, 1958.

Klatzo, I., Wisniewski, H., Smith, D. E.: Observations on penetration of serum proteins into the central nervous system. Prog. Brain Res. 15:73–88, 1965.

Kornecki, E., Ehrlich, Y. H.: Neuroregulatory and neuropathological actions of the ether-phospholipid platelet-activating factor. Science 240:1792–1794, 1988.

Koto, A., Rosenberg, G., Zingesser, L. H., Horoupian, D., Katzman, R.: Syndrome of normal pressure hydrocephalus: Possible relation to hypertensive and arteriosclerotic vasculopathy. J. Neurol. Neurosurg. Psychiatry 40:73–79, 1977.

Levin, E. G., Loskutoff, D. J.: Regulation of plasminogen activator production by cultured endothelial cells. Ann. NY Acad. Sci. 401:184–194, 1982.

Levine, S.: Anoxic–ischemic encephalopathy in rats. Am. J. Pathol. 36:1–17, 1960.

Levy, D. E., Brierley, J. B., Silverman, D. G., Plum, F.: Brief hypoxia–ischemia initially damages cerebral neurons. Arch. Neurol. 32:450–456, 1975.

Long, D. M., Hartmann, J. F., French, L. A.: The response of experimental cerebral edema to glucosteroid administration. J. Neurosurg. 24:843–854, 1966.

Lundberg, N.: Continuous recording and control of ventricular fluid pressure in neurosurgical practice. Acta. Psychiatr. Scand. [suppl.] 149:36, 1960.

Marshall, L. F., Smith, R. W., Rauscher, L. A., Shapiro, H. M.: Mannitol dose requirements in brain-injured patients, J. Neurosurg. 48:169–172, 1978.

Marshall, L. F., Smith, R. W., Shapiro, H. M.: The outcome with aggressive treatment in severe head injury. Part I: The significance of intracranial pressure monitoring. J. Neurosurg. 50:20–25, 1979.

McIntosh, T. K., Faden, A. I., Bendall, M. R., Vink, R.: Traumatic brain injury in the rat: Alterations in brain lactate and pH as characterized by ^{1}H and ^{31}P nuclear magnetic resonance. J. Neurochem. 49:1530–1540, 1987.

McKissock, W., Richardson, A., Taylor, J.: Primary intracerebral hemorrhage: A controlled trial of surgical and conservative treatment in 189 unselected cases. Lancet. 2:221–226, 1961.

Milhorat, T. H., Clark, R. G., Hammock, M. K., McGrath, P. P.: Structural, ultrastructural, and permeability changes in the ependyma and surrounding brain favoring equilibration in progressive hydrocephalus. Arch. Neurol. 22:397–407, 1970.

Miller, J. D.: Volume and pressure in the craniospinal axis. Clin. Neurosurg. 22:76–105, 1975.

Norris, J. W., Pappius, H. M.: Cerebral water and electrolytes. Effect of asphyxia, hypoxia, and hypercapnia. Arch. Neurol. 23:248–258, 1970.

Olszewski, J.: Subcortical arteriosclerotic encephalopathy: Review of the literature on the so-called Binswanger's disease and presentation of 2 cases. World Neurology 3:359–375, 1962.

Panetta, T., Marcheselli, V. L., Braquet, P., Spinnewyn, B., Bazán, N. G.: Effects of a platelet-activating factor antagonist (BN 52021) on free fatty acids, diacylglycerols, polyphosphoinositides and blood flow in the gerbil brain: Inhibition of ischemia–reperfusion-induced cerebral injury. Biochem. Biophys. Res. Commun. 149:580–587, 1987.

Pappius, H. M., Gulati, D. R.: Water and electrolyte content of cerebral tissues in experimentally induced edema. Acta. Neuropathol. 2:451–460, 1963.

Paschen, W., Djuricic, B., Mies, G., Schmidt-Kastner, R., Linn, F.: Lactate and pH in the brain: Association and dissociation in different pathophysiological states. J. Neurochem. 48:154–159, 1987.

Plum, F., Posner, J. B., Alvord, E. C.: Edema and necrosis in experimental cerebral infarction. Arch. Neurol. 9:563–570, 1963.

Pullen, R. G. L., De Pasquale, M., Cserr, H. F.: Bulk flow of cerebrospinal fluid into brain in response to acute hyperosmolality. Am. J. Physiol. 253:F538–F545, 1987.

Pulsinelli, W. A., Brierley, J. B., Plum, F.: Temporal profile of neuronal damage in a model of transient forebrain ischemia. Ann. Neurol. 11:491–498, 1982.

Quindlen, E. A., Bucher, A. P.: Correlation of tumor plasminogen activator with peritumoral cerebral edema. A CT and biochemical study. J. Neurosurg. 66:729–733, 1987.

Rennels, M. L., Gregory, T. F., Blaumanis, O. R., Fujimoto, K., Grady, P. A.: Evidence for a "paravascular" fluid circulation in the mammalian central nervous system, provided by the rapid distribution of tracer protein throughout the brain from the subarachnoid space. Brain Res. 326:47–63, 1985.

Reulen, H. J., Tsuyumu, M., Tack, A., Fenske, A. R., Prioleau, G. R.: Clearance of edema fluid into cerebrospinal fluid. A mechanism for resolution of vasogenic brain edema. J. Neurosurg. 48:754–764, 1978.

Roblin, R., Young, P. L.: Dexamethasone regulation of plasminogen activator in embryonic and tumor-derived human cells. Cancer Res. 40:2706–2713, 1980.

Ropper, A. H.: Fundamental clinical aspects of increased intracranial pressure; monitoring and treatment. In Handbook of Critical Care Neurology and Neurosurgery. Henning, R. J., Jackson, D. L., eds. New York: Praeger, 1985:89–102.

Rosenberg, G. A., Kornfeld, M., Stovring, J., Bicknell, J. M.: Subcortical arteriosclerotic encephalopathy (Binswanger): Computerized tomography. Neurology 29:1102–1106, 1979.

Rosenberg, G. A., Kyner, W. T., Estrada, E.: Bulk flow of brain interstitial fluid under normal and hyperosmolar conditions. Am. J. Physiol. 238:42–49, 1980.

Rosenberg, G. A., Kyner, W. T., Estrada, E.: The effect of increased CSF pressure on interstitial fluid flow during ventriculocisternal perfusion in the cat. Brain Res. 232:141–150, 1982.

Rosenberg, G. A., Saland, L., Kyner, W. T.: Pathophysiology of periventricular tissue changes with raised CSF pressure in cats. J. Neurosurg. 59:606–611, 1983.

Rosenberg, G. A., Wolfson, L. I., Katzman, R.: Pressure-dependent bulk flow of cerebrospinal fluid into brain. Exp. Neurol. 60:267–276, 1978.

Ryder, H. W., Espey, F. F., Kimbell, E. D., Penka, E. J., Rosenauer, A., Podolsky, B., Evans, J. P.: The mechanism of the change in cerebrospinal fluid pressure following an induced change in the volume of the fluid space. J. Lab. Clin. Med. 41:428–435, 1953.

Sahar, A., Tsipstein, E.: Effects of mannitol and furosemide on the rate of formation of cerebrospinal fluid. Exp. Neurol. 60:584–591, 1978.

Schaeffer, B. E., Zadunaisky, J. A.: Stimulation of chloride transport by fatty acids in corneal epithelium and relation to changes in membrane fluidity. Biochim. Biophys. Acta. 556:131–143, 1979.

Siesjo, B. K., Wieloch, T.: Cerebral metabolism in ischaemia: Neurochemical basis for therapy. Br. J. Anaesth. 57:47–62, 1985.

Spinnewyn, B., Blavet, N., Clostre, F., Bazán, N., Braquet, P.: Involvement of platelet-activating factor (PAF) in cerebral post-ischemic phase in Mongolian gerbils. Prostaglandins 34:337–349, 1987.

Steingart, A., Hachinski, V. C., Lau, C., Fox, A. J., Diaz, F., Cape, R., Lee, D., Inzitari, D., Merskey, H.: Cognitive and neurologic findings in subjects with diffuse white matter lucencies on computed tomographic scan (leukoaraiosis). Arch. Neurol. 44:32–35, 1987a.

Steingart, A., Hachinski, V. C., Lau, C., Fox, A. J., Fox, H., Lee, D., Inzitari, D., Merskey, H.: Cognitive and neurologic findings in demented patients with diffuse white matter lucencies on computed tomographic scan (leukoaraiosis). Arch. Neurol. 44:36–39, 1987b.

Stern, W. E., Coxon, R. V.: Osmolality of brain tissue and its relation to brain bulk. Am. J. Physiol. 206:1–7, 1964.

Stocks, J., Dormandy, T. L.: The autoxidation of human red cell lipids induced by hydrogen peroxide. Br. J. Haematol. 20:95–111, 1971.

Suzuki, R., Yamaguchi, T., Kirino, T., Orzi, F., Klatzo, I.: The effects of 5-minute ischemia in Mongolian gerbils: I. Blood–brain barrier, cerebral blood flow, and local cerebral glucose utilization changes. Acta. Neuropathol. (Berl) 60:207–216, 1983a.

Suzuki, R., Yamaguchi, T., Li, C. L., Klatzo, I.: The effects of 5-minute ischemia in Mongolian gerbils: II. Changes of spontaneous neuronal activity in cerebral cortex and CAl sector of hippocampus. Acta. Neuropathol. (Berl) 60:217–222, 1983b.

Tans, J. T. J., Poortvliet, D. C. J.: Reduction of ventricular size after shunting for normal pressure hydrocephalus related to CSF dynamics before shunting. J. Neurol. Neurosurg. Psychiatry 51:521–525, 1988.

Tuhrim, S., Dambrosia, J. M., Price, T. R., Mohr, J. P., Wolf, P. A., Heyman, A., Kase, C. S.: Prediction of intracerebral hemorrhage survival. Ann. Neurol. 24:258–263, 1988.

Turrens, J. F., Crapo, J. D., Freeman, B. A.: Protection against oxygen toxicity by intravenous injection of liposome-entrapped catalase and superoxide dismutase. J. Clin. Invest. 73:87–95, 1984.

Usher, J. R., Epand, R. M., Papahadjopoulos, D.: The effect of free fatty acids on the thermotropic phase transition of dimyristoyl glycerophosphocholine. Chem. Phys. Lipids 22:245–253, 1978.

Van Harreveld, A., Collewijn, H., Malhotra, S. K.: Water, electrolytes and extracellular space in hydrated and dehydrated brains. Am. J. Physiol. 210:251–256, 1966.

Wallach, D., Pastan, I.: Stimulation of guanylate cyclase of fibroblasts by free fatty acids. J. Biol. Chem. 251:5802–5809, 1976.

Warrell, D. A., Looareesuwan, S., Warrell, M. J., Kasemsarn, P., Intaraprasert, R., Bunnag, D., Harinasuta, T.: Dexamethasone proves deleterious in cerebral malaria. A double-blind trial in 100 comatose patients. N. Engl. J. Med. 306:313–319, 1982.

Wasterlain, C. G., Posner, J. B.: Cerebral edema in water intoxication. I. Clinical and chemical observations. Arch. Neurol. 19:71–78, 1968.

Wasterlain, C. G., Torack, R. M.: Cerebral edema in water intoxication. II. An ultrastructural study. Arch. Neurol. 19:79–87, 1968.

Weiss, S. J., Peppin, G., Ortiz, X., Ragsdale, C., Test, S. T.: Oxidative autoactivation of latent collagenase by human neutrophils. Science 227:747–749, 1985.

Wise, B. L., Chater, N.: The value of hypertonic mannitol solution in decreasing brain mass and lowering cerebrospinal fluid pressure. J. Neurosurg. 19:1038–1043, 1962.

Yoshida, S., Abe, K., Busto, R., Watson, B. D., Kogure, K., Ginsberg, M. D.: Influence of transient ischemia on lipid-soluble antioxidants, free fatty acids and energy metabolites in rat brain. Brain Res. 245:307–316, 1982.

INDEX